OXFORD MEDICAL PUBLICATIONS

Violence in Health Care   362.11/SHE

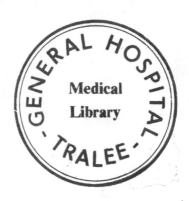

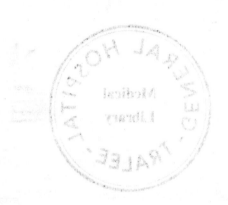

Violence in Health Care

A Practical Guide to Coping with Violence and Caring for Victims

Edited by

JONATHAN SHEPHERD

Professor of Oral and Maxillofacial Surgery
University of Wales College of Medicine

Oxford   New York   Tokyo
OXFORD UNIVERSITY PRESS
1994

Oxford University Press, Walton Street, Oxford OX2 6DP

Oxford   New York   Toronto
Delhi   Bombay   Calcutta   Madras   Karachi
Kuala Lumpur   Singapore   Hong Kong   Tokyo
Nairobi   Dar es Salaam   Cape Town
Melbourne   Auckland   Madrid
and associated companies in
Berlin   Ibadan

Oxford is a trade mark of Oxford University Press

Published in the United States
by Oxford University Press Inc., New York

A catalogue record for this book is available from the British Library

Library of Congress Cataloging in Publication Data
Shepherd, Jonathan.
Violence in health care: a practical guide to coping with violence
and caring for victims/Jonathan Shepherd.
Includes bibliographical references and index.
1. Medical personnel–Assaults against. 2. Violence in hospitals.
3. Victims of crimes–Services for. 4. Family violence.
5. Violence–Prevention. I. Title.
R727.2.S53   1994   362.1'1'0684–dc20   93–43592

ISBN 0 19 262157 2

Typeset by The Electronic Book Factory Ltd, Fife
Printed in Great Britain on acid-free paper by
Biddles Ltd, Guildford and King's Lynn

Preface

Violent behaviour is an important problem. Increasing numbers of victims, including many health professionals, seek support and treatment and need rehabilitation. It has become apparent that health-care workers are largely unaware of the background and circumstances of violence and of the needs of victims. These areas of expertise have been considered in the past to belong to the police and agencies such as Victim Support. However, three-quarters of violent crimes resulting in the need for medical treatment are not recorded by the police, from whom victim support agencies receive virtually all their referrals. Doctors, nurses, and other health-care workers have a responsibility to provide opportunities for wider support, and need to recognize their own vulnerability. The provision of health care in a violent society carries with it risks that need to be recognized.

Violence has become as much a public health issue as accidents, since both give rise to large numbers of deaths and injuries. There is a need for those who care for victims to appreciate causes, patterns, and the potential severity of injury, as well as the likely psychological and social sequelae.

It is a fact of life that violent behaviour is a feature of day-to-day clinical work in primary care, Accident and Emergency departments, and the home. There is a need for health-care workers to know how to cope with aggressive behaviour. The greater the extent of patient contact the greater the risk of assault. Junior staff at the outset of training are particularly vulnerable, for example, nurses, who have not had time to develop relationships with elderly patients.

A team of experts has been brought together to produce this handbook, which summarizes information relevant to those who treat victims and to those at risk of violence. Contributors also include psychiatrists, criminologists, a surgeon, a nurse, a lawyer, and a family practitioner who was assaulted and badly injured during a consultation. Because health care workers often meet victims of domestic and other intentional violence and their relatives, chapters are included which deal with these areas.

This wide-ranging handbook describes what it feels like to be a victim of violence and how best to get over the inevitable physical circumstances of violent crime, at-risk groups such as battered wives and delinquent young men, the epidemiology of violence, and the needs of the victims. A logical programme for the care of victims is presented, emphasizing interrelated physical, psychological, and psychiatric needs. The handbook also includes details and advice concerning applications for compensation from the Criminal Injuries Compensation Board and other agencies. Practical advice on the avoidance of violence is given, particularly in relation to home visits in high-crime areas, communication skills, clinic design, and liaison with community crime prevention initiatives. Advice is given on ways in which aggression can be dealt with.

Names and addresses of voluntary and statutory support agencies, with details of expertise, are included. The information given is not intended to be exhaustive, and those requiring more details should consult standard textbooks in criminology and related subjects.

I hope this book will help general practitioners, Accident and Emergency staff, hospital and community nurses and social workers, psychiatrists and clinical psychologists, surgeons, dentists, and other health-care workers who come into contact with the victims of violent crime not only to provide more informed and comprehensive treatment, but to know where to turn after attacks and aggression have been directed against themselves. Managers will also find this book useful because it describes ways in which safe working environments can be created, so that damaging civil actions by employees can be avoided. A list of addresses and telephone numbers of organizations, including trade unions, which provide help and advice in the event of injury or threat of injury will be an invaluable source of help for all health-care workers, including such diverse groups as pharmacists, ambulance staff, chiropractors, and receptionists..

I am very grateful to the organizations listed in the appendices for letting me have information about the services they offer.

Cardiff   J.P.S.
January 1994

Foreword

Helen Reeves, O.B.E.,
Director, Victim Support

After being concerned with crime throughout my career, first as a Probation Officer and then at Victim Support, I am only too well aware of the essential role which health care workers play in dealing with the aftermath of criminal violence. But too little information has been published about the specific needs of crime victims, and it is scattered through many different journals – so I am very pleased to welcome this new book on violent crime.

A series of research findings in recent years has highlighted the involvement of health care workers in the problems of crime. Karen Williams' Home Office study, *Community resources for victims of crime*, published in 1983, confirmed that in the absence of specialist services for victims of crime, help was most often sought from GPs. All too often, the effects of the crime had already been neglected and serious symptoms of anxiety or depression had already developed, for which medication, even if necessary to alleviate distress, was never going to be an adequate answer.

British Crime Surveys, introduced during the 1980s, confirmed the suspicions of many practitioners: that a high proportion of crime is not reported to the police, and that this includes many serious crimes of violence. The victims in many cases have been too fearful to seek help from the police, because of their anxiety that the involvement of the criminal justice process might increase their vulnerability to repeated attacks and harassment.

Victim Support's inter-agency Working Party on Domestic Violence and its demonstration project on racially motivated crime have confirmed the level of fear which exists, resulting in victims of some of the most serious crimes feeling unable to seek help with their problems. But the medical effects of injury and distress cannot be avoided, and help is sought from medical services who are then faced with important professional decisions as to how best to intervene.

More recently, attention has also been focused on the risks of violence to health care workers themselves when called to work with some of the more unstable members of the community. This newly identified problem produces additional problems and responsibilities for everyone in the health service as colleagues, managers, and employers.

Once again, we find that no social problem can be dealt with in isolation. Human behaviour, social relationships, and health are all inextricably linked. Equally, those of us responsible for dealing with the problems do not have to work in isolation. Many GPs and Accident & Emergency departments already enjoy close links with their local Victim Support, and Jonathan Shepherd has been energetic in making both the medical profession and Victim Support aware of the unmet needs. Everyone benefits, not least the victims, from the important opportunities thus provided for referral for help or advice and for shared training.

I welcome this valuable book, providing in a single volume the essentials which all health care workers should know about coping with the effects of violent crime. I hope that it will be widely read, and look forward to a closer working relationship between the health care professions and those of us who work with victims of crime.

Contents

8 Non-accidental injury of children 135

Dr Alan Emond, Consultant Community Paediatrician
Bristol Royal Hospital for Sick Children

9 The causes and prevention of offending, with special reference to violence 149

Professor David P. Farrington, Institute of Criminology
University of Cambridge

Names and addresses of voluntary and statutory support
agencies and their areas of expertise

1 Effects of assault on health-care professionals

Gillian Mezey and Jonathan Shepherd

Assaults on health-care staff are common, and are on the increase particularly in primary care settings and in the Accident and Emergency Department. Risk factors associated with assault at work include lack of trained staff, working in isolation, low staff levels, inadequate security, and situations where there is little active therapeutic activity involving the patients. Assaults are often precipitated by apparently trivial disputes over space or personal possessions – which may well have increased significance to individuals confined within a restricted space. In the United Kingdom, the Health Services Advisory Commission found that one in ten employees had suffered minor injuries as a result of being assaulted by a patient, and the under-reporting of incidents is widespread. Health workers identified as being at particularly high risk are ambulance staff, family practitioners working in deprived areas, nurses (particularly those in training), Accident and Emergency workers, and those caring for psychologically disturbed individuals, including the mentally handicapped.

Attacks arise for a variety of reasons: they may be instrumental, criminal, or malicious, or committed because of mental state, altered level of consciousness, or drug or alcohol intoxication, without intent or any prior planning on the part of the assailant. Assaults may be relatively minor or more serious, ranging from verbal abuse, intimidation, and physical or sexual harassment to physical or sexual assault. In the most extreme cases, physical injury or even the death of the victim may result.

Wherever health staff are in contact with the public, whether during the day or at night, or work within open facilities with free public access, they should be considered to be at risk. The Health and Safety at Work Act in 1974 imposed a statutory duty on Health Authorities to provide a safe working environment for their employees. However, health professionals are notoriously inaccurate in judging and predicting potential dangerousness. Assaults should be regarded as an occupational hazard of working as a health professional, particularly one exposed to high-risk situations or unpredictable patients.

THE EFFECTS OF ASSAULT ON THE VICTIM (Tables 1.1–1.3)

People assaulted at work tend to experience similar effects to those assaulted in the community, and have a right to expect similar consideration and access to treatment.

The impact of an assault on individuals and the health-care teams in which they work can be profound, and although a study of assaulted nurses found that 50 per cent denied any after-effects, other studies have remarked on the tendency of health workers to deny and minimize both the seriousness of the assaults and their physical and psychological impact. Reasons for not reporting violent incidents include the effort required, the fact that staff become inured to patient assault, and the view that being assaulted by a patient represents a performance failure. Telling the police about an assault is particularly unlikely, for fear that the disclosure of such information will be regarded as a breach of confidence.

The natural history of recovery from assault in health professionals is uncertain, because very few investigators have bothered to ask the victims themselves about the impact of their experience. The effects of violence depend on a number of factors, including the seriousness

---

Table 1.1 Psychological effects of assault

- Depression
- Guilt
- Loss of confidence
- Loss of sense of professional competence
- Increased feelings of vulnerability
- Self-doubts about capacity to continue
- Anger—unfocused or directed
- Irritability
- Generalized anxiety
- Decreased concentration

Table 1.2 Physical effects of assault

- Insomnia
- Nightmares
- Loss of or increased appetite
- Various physical complaints, such as:

  lethargy

  headaches

  muscle tension

  nausea, etc.
- Decreased sexual activity

Table 1.3 Behavioural effects (medium-term)

- Increased alcohol consumption
- Increased cigarette consumption
- Increased use of drugs to combat anxiety
- Increased startle response
- Absenteeism from work
- Avoidance of patient-contact
- Social withdrawal
- Loss of interest and involvement in work
- Phobic avoidance of reminders of assault

of the assault and the injuries sustained, the victim's personality, and the response of the victims' colleagues and social networks. Violence may result in emotional and behavioural changes, and can lead to alteration in the victims' relationships with colleagues and with their patients, and to altered attitudes to the workplace. Occasionally even apparently trivial assaults can result in a severe and prolonged response: the incident may trigger emotions associated with past episodes of violence, or may cause unresolved personal conflicts to surface. This response needs to be recognized and understood in, for example, family practitioners and nurses working in health centres in poor urban areas (see Chapter 2).

Psychological effects range from transient stress reactions lasting hours or days, to generalized depression and phobic anxiety and to specific prolonged reactions, including 'burnout' and post-traumatic stress disorder. Many victims of assault suffer from disrupted concentration, decreased efficiency in functioning at home or in the workplace, increased irritability, and exaggerated startle response (Table 1.5, p. 10). In the majority of cases, symptoms resolve within days or weeks; but prolonged distress may also occur.

The immediate response to an assault is generally a profound sense of helplessness. The normal reaction of an individual is to freeze, and this response, in the face of personal threat, is exacerbated by the constraints on health-care professionals that, however threatened and vulnerable they feel, they must never retaliate. They must not respond by attacking or striking the patient. Whatever the victims' instincts, it is the professionals' responsibility to control any anger they may feel and resist retaliating; indeed, not only to resist retaliating, but to continue to help and assist their 'assailants' in a therapeutic way. Unfortunately, this response sometimes includes 'denial' that the assault has taken place, and therefore increased likelihood of prolonged psychological distress.

Many victims experience a profound sense of shock and disbelief following an attack at work. Victims feel humiliated, and experience a loss of composure. They may feel outraged that they have been taken advantage of and that their identity as a health professional has been attacked and undermined. Fortunately, the majority of assaults by patients or their relatives do not lead to physical injury; but this means that the victim has no objective evidence of the experience and little obvious reason to feel hurt or distressed afterwards. The experience of assault is discrepant with the sort of experiences people hope for when they join the 'helping' professions. The experience of violence and being attacked does not, for most workers, enter into the expected general scheme of things. In a sense, health professionals assume that their 'uniform' – their identification as a helper – should confer on them an immunity from other people's aggression. Most health workers wish to be seen as 'good' people; and to respond to this 'goodness' with aggression seems undeserved and unfair.

MAKING SENSE OF VIOLENCE

A general response to misfortune is to attempt to 'make sense of it' in terms of what is already known and understood about the world and one's immediate environment. The disbelief many victims express is related to a failure to reconcile what has happened with a view of the hospital or the practice and its neighbourhood as a 'safe' environment. The 'just world' hypothesis, developed by Lerner in the 1930s, suggests that in a just world people 'get what they deserve and deserve what they get'. The victims of violence at work make sense of this in terms of what they may have done to have brought on or deserved such attacks, given that their status as health professionals should not in itself have led them to be victimized.

Individuals who have been assaulted often feel extremely vulnerable, and experience a loss of trust in people. This may be particularly damaging for primary care personnel who have developed long term relationships with their patients over many years. This loss of trust may spill over into their personal life, expressing itself as increased irritability and anger, which is suppressed at work. This can lead to more arguments with a partner, decreased tolerance of children, and existing on a 'short fuse'. Many workers find concentration is difficult after an assault. Concentration is often disrupted by ruminations over the assault along the lines of, 'Why did it happen?', 'If only . . .', 'What did I do wrong?', 'Why me?', and reliving the event in an attempt to find an explanation. An assault by a stranger in the street on the way to a home visit is clearly distressing; but then the street is often regarded as a dangerous place. The surgery or out-patient clinic, like the home, is usually regarded as a safe place; and therefore an attack can lead to the question of where an individual can really feel secure.

The experience of violence challenges a number of basic assumptions about personal safety and vulnerability, about the safety of the world around, and about the predictability of the future. It leads individuals to recognize their comparative helplessness and inability to control events. It leads victims to question their own responsibility for assaults, and gives rise to feelings of rage, distress, and impotence that a health professional could be attacked by someone seeking or receiving help. But also the victim frequently attributes the attack to some personal failure, and redirects feelings of anger inwards, in the form of guilt and self-blame. The victim needs to explain and make sense of the attack by attributing it to personal carelessness or lack of judgement in terms of 'How did I provoke this?' Self-blame can allow victims subsequently to regain a sense of control over future events: by changing what they do, they can increase their sense of control and reduce their fear of encountering further assaults. They may question how they can continue to treat people when their instinct is to run away or retaliate.

For some victims, it may be helpful to see attackers as being 'sick', unable to control their actions, and to attribute the violence to a disturbed mind rather than viewing it as a deliberate malevolent act. Nevertheless, many health workers see their own victimization as evidence of their own personal failure to care for the patient. In a study of assaulted doctors over half stated that they had acted in a provocative manner, and slightly more said they should have anticipated the assault. The majority of them denied and minimized the seriousness or significance of what had happened, and were reluctant to take any action. Another study of assaulted nurses found that most experienced anger, helplessness, and self-blame, but were unwilling to acknowledge the problem. The tendency of victims of assault at work to feel responsible for what has happened may be exacerbated by the unsympathetic and unsupportive response of their colleagues and social networks to their distress. The victims' professional and personal abilities are frequently brought into question by colleagues. A negative stereotype exists of the assaulted practitioner, often a view that he or she had 'asked for it', and victims may find themselves scapegoated by their non-assaulted colleagues. The less severe the assault the more the victim is blamed; female victims tend to be blamed more than men, while men and older people tend to be more critical of the assaulted employee. Blame and critical comments by other colleagues tend to be internalized by victims, and translated into feelings of guilt, self-doubt, and blame. There is clearly reluctance on all sides to acknowledge the random and arbitrary nature of victimization. Prediction of patient violence by professionals is notoriously unreliable; yet recognition of this fact challenges the professional's self-image of being in control. Care-givers may also find it uncomfortable to perceive themselves and to be perceived by others as in need of care and assistance, as being helpless and vulnerable rather than in control. However, this denial can be very destructive, as stress and low morale take their toll in feelings of inadequacy, isolation from peers, apathy, depression, and withdrawal. While the abusive patient is excused, the victimized health-professional is not only blamed, but often denied access to treatment.

LONG-TERM EFFECTS (Table 1.4)

Other specific responses to assault can be depression and anxiety, self-doubt, loss of self-confidence, and questioning one's own ability to interact in a therapeutic way with one's patients. Extreme fear and phobic anxiety may be expressed as various somatic complaints, including a dry mouth, tightness in the chest, palpitations, sweating, and agitation. Individuals may attempt to cope with feelings of anxiety and insomnia by increased use of alcohol and tranquillizing drugs. Guilt and self-blame in response to an assault are very common amongst assaulted workers. Indeed, it seems to be much more difficult to blame the assailant. More common is a feeling of resentment towards and a tendency to blame the 'boss', the health-service and one's colleagues, for failing to protect one. Sometimes of course, this may be the case, and assaults can be to some extent a reflection of neglect on the part of employers. Insomnia and decreased appetite may be experienced transiently, along with social withdrawal.

PHYSICAL EFFECTS OF ASSAULT

Fortunately, serious physical injury is infrequent following assaults to health-care professionals. However, because most violence is directed towards the head and face, most physical sequelae are obvious to friends, colleagues, and patients and may be interpreted as the results of fighting, domestic violence, or even drunkenness. Usually, attacks with fists or with blunt weapons close to hand, such as crockery or small items of furniture, are the cause of injury, so that lacerations are infrequent. To reduce the risk of injury, glassware and crockery used in health-centres, hospitals, and clinics should be manufactured from toughened (tempered) material. Tempered glassware is now widely available, and is often no more expensive

---

Table 1.4 Long-term effects

- Increased absenteeism → Resignation
- 'Burn out syndrome'
- Post-traumatic stress disorder

than untoughened products. Toughened tableware is much more resistant to breakage than other types, and, when it does break, tends to fragment into relatively harmless 'sugar lump' pieces. When lacerations do occur, then permanently disfiguring scars often result, despite the best suturing and repair techniques.

Blunt injuries of the face commonly cause bruising, particularly around the eye; but bruising is likely to affect any traumatized area. Bruising tends to move down the face as it resolves. Left-sided injuries are much more common than right-sided, because most assailants are right-handed. About 20 per cent of assaults which result in facial injuries give rise to broken facial bones. Broken noses, cheek-bones, and lower jaws are common in assault. A broken cheek-bone often gives rise to difficulty in chewing, numbness of the cheek and upper lip, double vision, and deformity, because the cheek-bone has been displaced inwards or downwards. This often requires an operation, after which most of the problems resolve; but the numbness, which occasionally lasts for months or even years, may be a particularly long-standing reminder of what has happened.

A broken nose gives rise to obvious deformity, and may require an operation to reduce it. After-effects may include change in facial appearance, difficulty with breathing, and increased likelihood of sinusitis. It is particularly important that these injuries are assessed by the appropriate specialist at an early stage, so that later complications are avoided.

The lower jaw is most often broken just below the jaw joint in front of the ear. Such an injury, which often requires no surgical intervention, gives rise to severe jaw stiffness, swelling in front of the ear, and alteration in the way the teeth meet. Such alterations in the way in which teeth meet together can be particularly noticeable and worrying, though in the case of these fractures the problem usually resolves without the need for an operation. The lower jaw can also break near the chin or at the angle of the jaw in the region of the wisdom tooth. These injuries require treatment more frequently, and may give rise to bleeding in the mouth, numbness of the lower lip, and the need for dental treatment to deal with any broken or chipped teeth.

All these injuries give rise to some facial swelling and at least temporary changes in appearance. The health-care worker will be unable to carry out normal work in these circumstances; but most facial swelling, whether caused by bruising or inflammation, usually disappears during the first two weeks after injury.

More severe injury, head injuries, and injuries of the hand are much less frequent than facial injury, but give rise to complications which need to be recognized just as much in health-care professionals as in others. Head injuries may give rise to long-term headaches, memory loss, and other problems, and early assessment and continuing care are important. The upper limb is often the most commonly affected area after the face. Some injuries can result from raising an arm to ward off blows or to prevent more serious injury to the face, head, or trunk. This may give rise to lacerations, which may include injuries to tendons and ligaments. Clearly, early advice is necessary in order that rehabilitation can take place as efficiently as possible; but it needs to be acknowledged that the incapacity associated with serious hand injury can be devastating to health-care professionals.

Continuing physical symptoms, however minor – and perhaps only comprising some transient lip numbness – are a constant reminder of the original trauma, and can act as a trigger to psychological symptoms. It is important that assessments of the effects of injury take place in a collaborative way, so that the physical and psychological effects are not divorced from each other, but are seen as interrelating.

BURNOUT SYNDROME

Burnout syndrome was a term devised in the 1970s to describe a psychological state arising in response to chronic stress experienced by health professionals, leading to disillusionment, inefficient functioning at work, psychosomatic complaints, absenteeism and eventually, leaving the service. Burnout often arises in response to a dissonance between the individuals' expectations of the job and external demands that often exceed capacity. Clearly, the experience of being assaulted at work adds to a sense of being devalued and not appreciated, and may increase the likelihood of developing burnout syndrome – although the presence of adequate support and the opportunity to ventilate feelings afterwards may prevent this (see Chapter 5).

POST-TRAUMATIC STRESS DISORDER (Table 1.5)

This is a specific syndrome which has been identified following major disasters, and violent crime such as an assault at the hands of a patient. The syndrome includes physical, behavioural, and emotional responses, and has two major components. These consist of re-experiencing the trauma in the form of daydreams, nightmares,

Table 1.5 Post-traumatic stress disorder

A: An event outside the range of usual experience
     —markedly distressing to almost everyone.

B: Re-experience of the traumatic event by
     (1) Recurrent and intrusive recollections
     (2) Recurrent distressing dreams
     (3) Acting or feeling 'as if the event was happening again'
     (4) Intense distress when exposed to events that
         symbolize or resemble the event

C: Persistent avoidance of stimuli associated with the
     trauma or numbing of responsiveness including
     (1) Efforts to avoid thoughts and feelings or
         activities associated with the trauma
     (2) Inability to recall aspects of the trauma
         Decreased interest in significant activities
         Feelings of detachment from others
         Restricted range of effect
         Sense of fore-shortened future

D: Persistent feelings of increased arousal include
     Insomnia, anger outbursts, poor concentration,
     hypervigilance, exaggerated startle response,
     exaggerated reactivity when reminded of the event.

E: Duration of at least one month

and flashbacks to the assault or other disaster; and avoidance symptoms, such as avoiding situations and people that are reminiscent of the original trauma. Although assaults affecting health workers are in the main, not life-threatening, it is important to recognize that post-traumatic stress disorder can be experienced following even relatively trivial attacks, particularly those which are perceived as life-threatening at the time.

The experience of avoidance symptoms is of particular relevance to health workers, and affects their ability to function at work after assault. They are likely to experience high levels of anxiety, particularly in association with any situation that reminds them of or is similar to the original attack. The health worker may cope with these distressing feelings by avoiding the patient that has assaulted them, and this avoiding behaviour may include refusing to nurse the patient, requesting transfer, or going off sick. Such avoidance behaviour is then reinforced and rewarded as anxiety levels go down;

and, eventually, this situation may lead to the health worker's taking prolonged absences from work. Their absence will then make it more difficult for them to face up to the feared situation again, and this will lead to a further loss of self-confidence in their ability to function professionally. Prolonged absenteeism may eventually result in the worker's deciding to leave work altogether.

Compensation awards following an assault to health-care professionals are rare, though injury insurance is increasingly one of the benefits of belonging to a defence organization or trade union (see Appendix). However, most health workers who are assaulted are not seeking high financial reward. Compensation can be something as simple as an apology from the perpetrator, expressions of care and concern from senior staff, (particularly managers and clinical directors), and acknowledgement of the individual's distress. Occasionally, the victim may feel very angry – particularly when the assailant is a psychiatric patient, when the worker may feel that the patient has been allowed to get away with it simply because of his or her mental disorder. Assaulted staff often express strong feelings that the patient is, in fact, not ill and is simply feigning illness, that he or she is in control of his or her actions, and that he or she should be prosecuted, as in the normal course of events. But in fact, the prosecution of psychiatric patients is extremely rare, partly because of the reluctance of management to support claimants and, partly, because of the reluctance of the police to press charges.

2 Attacks on doctors and nurses

Stefan Cembrowicz and Susan Ritter

In common with the escalation of violent crime in Western society as a whole, aggressive incidents against GPs are also on the increase. In one survey 10 per cent of GPs had been assaulted, and 5 per cent threatened with a weapon. In another survey, 11 per cent of West Midlands GPs had been assaulted and 91 per cent had experienced verbal abuse. In London in 1987 11 per cent of GPs experienced an attack. A recent study has identified female nurses as most at risk of violence in the Accident and Emergency Department, and has found that receptionists are generally at low risk.

Anxiety about violence and personal abuse is often at the front of the minds of health-care professionals, and young women general practitioners have described clinics where several abusive, threatening patients have been seen using emotive terms like 'dread', 'cringe', and 'guilt'. GPs are sometimes assaulted or threatened if drugs are not prescribed.

It is clear that health-care professionals are subject to a good deal of violence and aggression, though, as yet, the extent is largely unquantified and the causes unexplained. Although a survey of violence to NHS staff suggests that staff in some institutions are more at risk than community staff, doctors and other health-care professionals working in the community are facing an increasing number of aggressive and violent assaults. For obvious reasons, these incidents are better prevented than experienced. The guidelines for prevention set out in this chapter are based on general principles and heuristics (rules-of-thumb). Much more research is needed before particular interventions can be definitively recommended over others. Unfortunately, the results of research from one kind of setting (for example, a mental hospital ward) cannot be applied to a different setting (for example, a patient's home); theoretical models are often oversimplified; and myths are easily perpetuated with little or no evidence. These reservations must be applied to any recommendations about the management of violence in health-care settings.

A threat of force against a doctor, nurse, or other health professional without legal justification represents an assault. To use force,
even if it amounts in the end to the lightest touch, constitutes battery.
Assault and battery are criminal offences, and victims can be awarded
compensation under civil law (see Chapter 6).

Although it is very clear when an assault has taken place, the
position of the victim is not necessarily clear in relation to the police.
Many medical and ancillary staff are uncertain about their rights, and
may be reluctant on ethical grounds, because of guilt, fear, or denial
of the severity of an incident, to pursue a patient through the courts.
Actual or grievous bodily harm, where the victim has been injured,
is more likely to be dealt with by the police, though of course
incidents first need to be reported. Minor injuries or threats are less
likely to be dealt with by the police. Pursuing private prosecution
presents many problems for staff, whether legal, financial, or ethical.
It is incumbent on employers, therefore, to have satisfactory systems
of preventing violence where possible, to support staff who have
been victims, and to learn from these incidents. These systems
will need to include formal liaison procedures with the local police.
Staff must always be encouraged by their employers to co-operate
with any police action after an assault. Otherwise, there will be an
implication that violence directed against health workers is somehow
acceptable.

CAUSES OF AGGRESSION DIRECTED AGAINST
HEALTH-CARE WORKERS

Explanation of violent behaviour includes socially mediated factors
and those which assume the presence of organic changes in the brain.
The various causes are separated here for the sake of explanation, but
it is important to remember that the psychotic or brain-damaged person is not immune to personal crises, and may be more susceptible
than other people to stressful relationships (see Chapter 4).

Behavioural crisis

Although violent incidents involving health-care staff may be a
result of mental or physical illness, or of deliberate criminal acts,
many incidents do not fit into these categories, and may be better
understood in terms of 'behavioural crises'. A behavioural crisis
has been defined as a response to a life event and associated
stress. Dramatic changes in behaviour can result, with damaging
consequences if the crisis is beyond the person's coping resources.

The most destructive violent event recorded in one study of violence concerned a middle-aged man who was distraught and angry after his father had died in an ambulance on the way to hospital after a coronary thrombosis. He felt that medical and ambulance staff were at fault. In these circumstances, crisis intervention is a management process aimed at:

- easing pain and stress;
- mobilizing the patient's own resources; and
- mobilizing outside resources.

The characteristics of a behavioural crisis include:

- confusion, upsetting emotions, and loss of abilities;
- anxiety, which may be immobilizing;
- preoccupation with physical symptoms; and
- feelings of helplessness, frustration, and anger.

This view of crisis assumes that anger may be displaced inwards, causing depression, withdrawal, and the wish for self-harm, or outwards, causing hostility and aggression. Patients experiencing these feelings tend to welcome calm, firm help to bring structure to their emotional chaos. People are particularly vulnerable at times of change in their lives, such as puberty, job or housing changes, marital insecurity, the menopause, and retirement.

Behavioural crises may resolve through:

- physical harm to self (including suicide attempts);
- physical harm to others (assault or family or child abuse);
- escape via alcohol;
- psychotic behaviour;
- running away; or
- inappropriate behaviour – petty crime (including shoplifting) and calls for help via the emergency services.

Crisis intervention

It is important to remember that during such a crisis, health-care staff may be dealing with:

- the person experiencing the crisis;
- secondary clients (concerned family and friends); and
- other carers (social workers, priests, teachers).

Both the person's own resources and those of other carers need to be mobilized in order to help resolve the crisis.

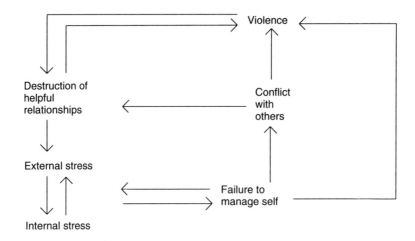

Diagram to show cycle of violence, stress, and failure to manage self and relationships.

Cycle of violence, stress, and failure to manage self and relationships

In this model, the vulnerable individual is likely to have had lifelong difficulties with relationships, often being subjected to contradictory pressures in childhood, such as being told by father to respect mother though he himself regularly beats her up when he is drunk (see Chapter 9). In such circumstances the child will have special difficulties in making helpful relationships outside the home, and will often be in conflict with both family and other people. The helper of someone who has repeated experiences of failure in relationships must be especially careful not to promise more than can be delivered, must be scrupulous about adhering to agreements, and must be prepared for apparently irrational attacks of blame and recrimination, which can explode into violence if responded to in kind.

Assertiveness versus aggression

Asserting oneself in a difficult situation involves avoiding the behavioural extremes of aggression and passivity. An aggressive response on the part of a health worker to an angry or complaining person increases the risk of further escalation through anger being met with anger. Passive people, however, may find hostile criticism particularly stressful, and feel victimized and resentful. Losing control of one's temper leads to the risks of over-reacting and triggering a violent episode. Yet a passive response to an angry patient may risk increasing his or her anger, as the response may be interpreted as a refusal to answer criticisms. Assertiveness, like other social skills, has to be learned. It means expressing one's own needs and wishes calmly and clearly while enabling the other person to present his or her own position, in order to find common ground for agreement. A health professional whose self-esteem is low, or who has learned that aggression generally forces compliance in others, will not have much incentive to learn assertiveness skills.

However, for health-care staff, assertiveness is increasingly recognized as an important part of communications skills, valuable not only when dealing with angry and complaining patients, but also when managing personnel and negotiating with managers.

Episodic dyscontrol

Some people are thought to be susceptible to bouts of uncontrollable rage, associated with evidence of minimal brain dysfunction. Episodic dyscontrol has also been reported in women during the days preceding menstruation. Such people can usually distinguish between 'normal' anger and such an episode, which can sometimes lead to serious injury to self or others.

Social learning theory

It has been argued that much can be understood and predicted about aggressive behaviour if the social context is known. Particular settings, such as football-fan or gun clubs, may be expected to reinforce specific behaviours. As long as these behaviours occur in this context they cause little social concern; but a football fan who behaves in a suburban residential street as he or she does on the terraces is likely to be labelled a hooligan. The gun-user who widens the context of weapon-use from club to the home is likely to be labelled as weird and aggressive. Aggression may be a product of reciprocal influences within individuals and the society with which they interact. Aggressive behaviour is likely to be reinforced by compliance in the people to whom it is directed. Other kinds of 'behaviour feedback' reinforce different as well as similar behaviours, so that the expression of aggression is modified by social as well as by internal experience. It has been suggested that a problem-solving approach can help individuals find constructive solutions to adversity. However, extreme emotional arousal prevents calm thinking, so that prevention and reduction of arousal in aggressive people must be a primary aim.

Prediction of violence and risk assessment

One of the best predictors of violent behaviour is a history of violent actions. However, very often health-care staff must deal with people whose history they do not know, attempting to provide help in the context of a relationship between strangers, which often involves early intrusions into areas of patients' lives that would normally be kept private. Moreover, even mental health professionals do not seem to be especially skilled at predicting the dangerousness of individuals.

In these circumstances, it is important to use a belt-and-braces approach, by attending to the role of environmental and organizational factors in preventing violence, by training staff to intervene as rapidly and as effectively as possible when a violent incident occurs, and by providing comprehensive support for staff who may be stressed both by the need to maintain high standards and the feelings of self-blame which usually result from involvement with a violent person.

PREVENTIVE STRATEGIES

Aspects of liaison procedures with police

Social contact with neighbourhood police officers who work in areas served by practices, clinics, and hospitals establishes a friendly relationship with known individuals. This will facilitate rapid and appropriate action when a member of staff needs help. Community constables or other officers can be encouraged to drop in on premises from time to time for a cup of tea. Regular review of premises by the local crime-prevention officer allows staff and police to get to know each other. Joint training sessions on skills such as anger-management and assertiveness, and on issues such as sexism or racism help staff and police to understand each other's points of view, professional difficulties, and pressures. More formal and regular meetings are necessary in order to monitor violent and other incidents, to review procedures, and to evaluate the quality of the liason itself. Some geographical areas have business-watch as well as neighbourhood-watch schemes.

Design of the workplace

Design of premises can play an important part in preventing violence to health-care workers. Prevention of violent episodes should be approached as thoroughly as the prevention of other health problems and hazards, such as the spread of infection. Much can be done to reduce the occurrence of violence by paying attention to how tasks are performed. The working environment is a major factor, though it should not be considered in isolation. Staff safety should always be considered at the design stage of any health-service building project, in consultation with those who will be using the premises. The objective is 'homely, non-threatening, security-conscious premises'. Consideration should be given to the ease with which the layout of premises and the activities of staff can be seen from outside by potential attackers, especially in darkness when lights are on. Conversely, the exterior of buildings needs to be well-lit, with lights in the parking area and along any paths leading to entrances. Closed circuit television, with a display of monitors in the reception area, may be a useful investment in some areas. A variety of computerized systems are available which link personal alarms with room alarms and indicators, centrally controlled by a computer which will automatically record and print out details of an incident as soon as an alarm is triggered. However, it is invariably human skills which prevent violence in the first place.

Human factors as they interact with design factors

Attempts to shelter reception staff behind heavy screening are no substitute for training them in interpersonal and interviewing skills, reviewing their work processes, and supporting them with an upgrading training programme. In general practice, for instance, the telephonist is often the first person to make contact with the patient. Each practice has its own system for message-handling, usually established by custom and the local working environment. For example, in some areas, many calls are received via call-boxes, and it is unrealistic to expect patients to wait for a call to be returned; whereas in other areas most patients will have a telephone. In the latter case, for example, it is possible to ring back and authenticate calls if necessary.

Telephone calls provide many opportunities for misunderstandings, hostility, and aggression to develop. A single-case analysis of an emergency call to an ambulance service by the son of a woman who suffered a respiratory collapse has been used in order to demonstrate the points at which an apparently orderly procedure can break down in the presence of callous and rigid staff attitudes and an agitated inarticulate caller.

A formal telephone drill will establish which calls should take priority. Well-trained and empathizing telephonists can help to

minimize patients' frustration by taking basic details efficiently and
deciding on each phone call's priority.

*Examples of classification of phone calls by type and priority of con-
tact needed*

1. *Contact doctor at once*
   These are calls about sudden medical emergencies: where there is
   talk of difficulty in breathing, collapse, chest-pain, bleeding, etc.
2. *Contact doctor at end of present consultation, having taken the
   number*
   These are calls where a visit may be needed.
3. *Contact doctor at end of surgery*
   These are calls for advice.
4. *Contact another team member, such as the practice nurse or social
   worker (immediately or later)*
   These are calls needing other team services.
5. *Contact appropriate receptionist for appointments, results of tests,
   other enquiries*
   These are administrative calls for appointments, results, and other
   enquiries.
6. *Personal calls*
   Family members: put through at once.
   Friends and other enquiries: take details for doctor to call back.

Complaints procedures

Many complaints against health-care staff arise not just from clinical
issues but from failures of communication. Maintaining sound clinical standards is of course vital; but providing a good service implies
more than this. Articulate patients who are dissatisfied may express
themselves via an immediate verbal complaint or a subsequent
written one. Less articulate people may not be able to use verbal
or written complaints as an outlet, and so may become increasingly
frustrated and even violent. Dealing with the consequences (which
can be psychological, physical, and even legal) is always unpleasant.
It is far preferable to deal with dissatisfied patients at an early stage
than to undergo a complaints procedure hearing or even an assault.
The arrangements for making informal or formal complaints about
family practitioner services are cumbersome, lengthy, and difficult
for both parties involved.

Striving to deliver services both efficiently and effectively at
both the clinical and personal levels can help prevent patients'
dissatisfaction, whether in the form of a minor grumble, a formal

complaint, or even an angry outburst. In the community, it may be possible to intercept grievances and remedy dissatisfaction by:

- using a suggestion box in the waiting-room;
- establishing a Patient Participation Group; and
- using the Practice Pamphlet to invite comments and complaints, and to direct them to a named team member: for example, a senior partner, practice manager, or senior receptionist.

In NHS hospitals, Department of Health guidelines resulting from the Hospital Complaints Act (1985) provide for a senior member of management to be responsible for dealing with patients' complaints. In general, if a patient complains verbally, he or she must be listened to carefully, and notes must be made of the details for later review. Because a reasonable complaint may be exaggerated, especially if patients feel that they are not being listened to, it is important not to get drawn into an argument, however unreasonable the grievance may at first appear. A written complaint needs an immediate and personal response. All complaints must be taken seriously. It will help to discuss any complaint with colleagues, preferably in team meetings, so that procedures can be reviewed in order to see whether there is any room for improvement.

In the event of a formal complaint, advice must be sought immediately from a Protection Society or other professional organization. All correspondence needs to be copied and discussed with a professional representative before replies are made.

Training

Staff training is essential for the smooth running of any health facility, so that face-to-face work with patients is impeded as little as possible by non-clinical issues. Sound staff-development policies and appraisal and supervision procedures provide the basis for an all-round competence in interpersonal skills, which in its turn is the basis for the variety of other specific skills of the individual staff member, whether doctor, dentist, health visitor, receptionist, or community psychiatric nurse.

Training for coping with violence can only be effective if it is embedded in a management structure which delegates the necessary authority to, say, a group or committee for the prevention and management of violent behaviour, which meets monthly and has a multiprofessional membership. This committee will approve and recommend policies and procedures; will make recommendations to professional and educational training committees; will review all violent incidents; and will make recommendations to clinical teams. Examples of relevant committees are a Nursing Professional Advisory Committee, a Health and Safety Committee, and a Joint Staff Consultative Committee.

Policies will make it mandatory for all staff to respond in an emergency; but this response will vary with the setting and the staff available. The policy will also specify the physical restraint techniques that are permissible; will identify the staff who have training responsibilities; and will state the kind and amount of initial and refresher training to be undertaken by staff. It is essential that this kind of policy structure protects staff who work in areas where violence and aggression are apt to occur. Nurses who agree to practise without these safeguards not only put themselves at risk, but they also fail to comply with Section 10 of the UKCC Code of Professional Conduct, which deals with safe standards of practice.

Restraint of violent people

At the present time, opinion is divided about whether 'Control and Restraint' by small teams is preferable to immobilization by larger teams or to mechanical restraint. On ethical grounds mechanical restraint has largely been discarded in the UK, although its use is widespread in Europe and the USA. A hospital or other health-care facility must decide whether it will use either Control and Restraint or Immobilization by a number of staff, and provide training for staff in one or the other method.

Training for restraint

An example of the kind of training that is now available for health-care professionals has been devised at Friern Barnet Hospital in North London. A variety of short courses have been developed from the Home Office-based Control and Restraint training, which was originally organized for the prison service and special hospitals. The Continuing Education Department is responsible for offering courses to ancillary staff such as receptionists and porters, longer courses for general clinical staff, and specialized courses for staff working in the community, primary-care settings and accident and emergency departments. These courses have much to teach nurses and family practitioners, whether doctors or dentists.

The techniques for dealing physically with violence which have been found to be most useful for nurses are the 'breakaway' techniques taught in Home Office-approved Control and Restraint courses. Over five days of initial training, nurses receive theoretical material dealing with the origins of violence and aggression; are exposed to aggressive behaviours; learn verbal and non-verbal responses to aggression; and practise the breakaway manoeuvres. It is important that these courses are run by Home Office-approved instructors: that is, that physical intervention techniques are not 'cascaded' by course participants. Instructors return regularly for refresher courses, and will in turn provide refresher courses for staff. Among the reasons for ensuring that techniques are learned in a controlled way is to reduce the chance that potential aggressors may learn them and apply them against staff.

Insurance

Insurance policies are now available which specifically cover injuries resulting from assault both for doctors and other staff (see Appendix I for details). However, it is necessary to check the small print on existing policies, as staff may find that they currently have little cover.

MANAGING AGGRESSION AND VIOLENT BEHAVIOUR

Body language

Non-verbal cues communicate a good deal about how people are feeling, and can give warning signals of increasing anxiety, tension, and anger. Few people are able to become violent without non-verbal warning signals. It is important to look out for:

- rapid breathing;
- clenched fists and teeth;
- flared nostrils;
- flushing
- loud talking or chanting;
- restless, repetitive movements; and
- pacing, gesticulating, and violent gestures, for example pointing.

Staff need to recognize their own body-language response to these signals. It is all too easy to respond unconsciously to a hostile stance in a way that increases interpersonal tension before a word has been spoken.

When talking to angry people:

- Pay close attention to them, and stand just outside their personal space – slightly out of arm's reach. If possible, stand on their non-dominant side (usually the side a wristwatch is worn or the hair parted).

- Use a quiet, and calm, but determined manner.
- Use calm body language: relaxed posture, hands open, attentive expression.
- Avoid staring eye contact.
- Avoid pointing at or touching angry people, or entering their personal space.

Arousal rating

An arousal rating scale has been devised for use in studies of assaults on staff in locked wards. Speech, activity/posture, and interpersonal distance can be rated. If two of the three variables of the arousal rating scale change, concern is justified, and defensive action may need to be taken. The simplicity of the scale makes it easy to memorize, and thus easy to use as a rapid assessment tool in areas where violent patients tend to be present.

General guidelines for preventing and managing violence

Action	Rationale
1. Don't be a loner.	1. If other staff do not know where you are or what you are doing, they will be unable to help if you run into difficulties.
2. Err on the side of anticipating aggression and potential violence.	2. (a) So that help is ready before a person actually becomes violent. (b) So that you can take advice before having to act. (c) To allow yourself time before tackling a problem.
3. Try to keep a balance between maintaining privacy for a patient and being isolated with a potentially violent person.	3. (a) So that you will not be cornered. (b) So that other staff can find you easily in case of trouble.
4. Always be courteous to clients and patients whatever their behaviour: conveying attentiveness; introducing yourself; remembering their names; attempting to identify and acknowledge concerns; appearing relaxed and non-aggressive yourself; and speaking quietly but audibly.	4. (a) People who are worried about themselves (or about a friend or relative) are much less likely to tolerate perceived discourtesy. (b) Failure to explain delays or queues can be interpreted as discourtesy or as dismissing clients' perceptions of their problems.

Action	Rationale
	(c) If you appear calm and confident it will help to calm the other person.
	(d) It is discourteous to shout or call across a room, and infringes privacy.
5. When first approaching patients, greet them by saying 'Good Morning' or similar words, and start any enquiry by using neutral or non-directive techniques for eliciting information: for example, 'Would you like to tell me how we can help you?'	5. (a) To convey a sense of normal social interaction. (b) To avoid provoking an anxious person.
6. Identify any signs of arousal in clients, such as a dry mouth, dilated pupils, sweating, rapid breathing, and a fast pulse.	6. Although these are not exclusively signs of anxiety or anger, they may alert you to a potentially aggressive response.
7. When giving an aggressive person information about their condition or treatment, do so in terms of suggestion rather than instruction.	7. (a) To avoid antagonizing him or her further. (b) So that you can repeat the explanation without appearing to lecture the person. (c) To allow you to see whether you are being understood.
8. Ensure that there is a system by which you can instantly summon help, for example alarm buttons in rooms and personal alarms.	8. (a) So that you can feel as well as appear calm and confident. (b) So that regular attenders get the message that aggression will not be tolerated.
9. Ensure that 'shop-front' staff such as receptionists receive appropriate training in interpersonal skills.	9. So that they do not unwittingly antagonise patients.
10. Ensure that 'shop-front' staff can ask health-care staff for advice as they need it.	10. So that potential problems can be anticipated and dealt with promptly.

Action

11. Ensure that 'shop-front' staff are not obliged to carry out tasks for which they are not qualified: for example, to assess the nature and severity of a person's condition.

12. Ensure that you are familiar with your department's policies and procedures for the prevention and management of violence.

13. Ensure that all new staff are thoroughly familiar with the geographical layout of the premises in which they will be working.

14. Arrange furniture in clinical areas in such a way that the staff member is nearer the door than the patient.

15. Ensure that you report and document all violent incidents.

16. Ensure that you are familiar with patterns of violence in your department.

17. Keep any jewellery, badges, pens, and scissors secure.

18. Keep all areas clean and tidy, and ensure that potential weapons like glassware, vases, etc. are sturdy and fixed.

19. Maintain good relations with the local police by identifying a liaison person; by having joint training sessions; and by agreeing joint policies.

Rationale

11. Patients can be distressed and irritated by having to explain their problems to a series of different and unidentified people.

12. So that you know what training you can expect and can apply it correctly.

13. (a) So that escape routes can be memorized.

(b) So that they will not allow themselves to be cornered.

14. So that it is always possible to escape if necessary.

15. So that resources can be allocated on the basis of accurate records.

16. So that you are prepared at times of risk.

17. To avoid injury in case you have to intervene physically with an aggressive person.

18. (a) Neglected, dirty or soiled surroundings and equipment do not inspire confidence, and may contribute to patients' hostility.

(b) If patients become violent they may seize any nearby object to use as a weapon.

19. (a) So that the police will come promptly when they are called.

(b) So that they will know the staff in the department and can work co-operatively with them.

(c) So that violent people can easily be dealt with in the criminal justice system when necessary.

Do's and Don'ts when facing an angry patient

DO	**DON'T**
• Recognize your own mood and feelings	• Meet anger with anger.
• Use calming body language.	• Raise your voice, point, stare.
• Put yourself in the patient's shoes: he or she may be anxious or afraid, as well as angry.	• Appear to lecture the patient.
• Be prepared to apologize if necessary.	• Threaten any intervention unless you are prepared to use it — immediately; — effectively; and — in safety.
• Assert yourself appropriately.	• Make the patient feel trapped or cornered.
• Allow people to 'get things off their chest'.	• Feel that you have to win the argument.

Common problems of aggressive behaviour

Problem	**Action**	**Rationale**
1. A patient or one of his or her relatives is verbally aggressive towards you.	1. (a)*Think*: 'This is an unfamiliar and stressful situation for this person, who may normally be able to be assertive without being aggressive.	1. (a) To use thinking time as a pause before acting on the problem. *And,* to put yourself in the other person's shoes. *And,* in order not to respond with hostility.
	(b) Behave calmly and in a relaxed way.	(b) By appearing calm, you encourage the other person to calm down.
	(c) Ensure that at least one colleague is aware of your situation.	(c) So that you can get help quickly if necessary.

Problem	**Action**	**Rationale**
1. A patient or one of his or her relatives is verbally aggressive towards you (*cont'd*).	(d) *Say*: 'I am sure that if you explain the problem to me I can find a way of helping you.'	(d) To convey that you are in control, and your confidence that the problem can be resolved.
	(e) Keep an eye on whether the person is becoming more or less tense.	(e) To decide what other interventions will be necessary.
	(f) Offer the person a seat while he or she talks to you.	(f) Sitting down is less compatible with a physical attack than standing up.
	(g) Keep at least an arm and a half's distance between you and the person	(g) So that he or she cannot hit you.
2. A patient or relative complains about another member of staff.	2. *Think*: 'My colleagues are busy and may have overlooked this patient's problem.	2. So that you pause before acting. Pursuing colleagues with recriminations will not address the complaint and will antagonize other staff.
	(b) *Think*: 'One of my colleagues may be dealing with this'.	(b) Anxious people often ask different staff the same question.
	(c) *Say*: 'I will find out for you exactly what is happening. I will either come back and let you know myself, or one of my colleagues will. Is that all right?'	(c) So that you make it clear that you are in control of the situation and that you take the complaint seriously.

Problem	Action	Rationale
2. A patient or relative complains about another member of staff (*cont'd*).	(d) Do immediately what you have undertaken to do.	(d) Once people have complained and feel that they have been ignored they may feel that they have to resort to violence.
3. You are criticized by a patient or his or her relative.	3. (a) *Think*: 'This person does not realize that by criticizing me he or she makes me appear incompetent in front of other patients and my colleagues.'	3. (a) So that you can respond neutrally and calmly to the person's needs without feeling aggrieved yourself *and* to give yourself a pause before acting.
	or	
	(b) *Think*: 'OK, I've made a mistake, but that does not make me a bad nurse.'	
	(c) *Say*: 'I apologize for . . . (for example, 'the delay') How can I help you?'	The reality of the situation is that the person wishes for some kind of help.
4. A patient becomes hostile and resistive during a procedure.	4. (a) *Think*: 'Because this is an uncomfortable and rather painful procedure, it is difficult for this person to be calm.'	4. (a) To give yourself a pause before responding.
	(b) Stop what you you are doing, if possible, and say 'Tell me what is wrong and I will try to put it right.'	(b) To encourage the patient to use words to express his or her feelings, rather than to act.

Problem	Action	Rationale
4. A patient becomes hostile and resistive during a procedure. (*cont'd*).	(c) Before and during any procedure, explain clearly and fully to the patient what is involved, how long it will take, and whether it will hurt.	(c) So that the patient can give informed consent to the treatment. *And* so that you remind the patient that he or she understands that there might be some pain or discomfort.
5. You have been seized round the neck from behind.	5. (a) Shout loudly for help.	5. (a) To surprise your assailant.
	(b) Grasp your assailant's little fingers and pull them outwards and forwards.	(b) To break the grip. *And* to extend the person's arms, thus preventing him or her from choking you.
6. Your tie or hair is being pulled.	6. (a) Shout loudly for help.	6. (a) To surprise your assailant.
	(b) Grasping the person's wrists, pull his or her hands towards you.	(b) To relax the tension on your hair or tie.
7. You have been seized around the neck by a person in front of you.	7. (a) Shout loudly for help.	7. (a) To surprise your assailant.
	(b) Cross your wrists in front of your neck, duck your head, and squat suddenly.	(b) To break the grip. *And* to protect your face as you duck.
8. You are being approached by a person holding a blunt object.	8. (a) Shout loudly for help.	8. (a) To surprise your assailant.

Problem	Action	Rationale
8. You are being approached by a person holding a blunt object. (*cont'd*).	(b) Remain facing the person while backing away.	(b) So that you cannot be attacked from behind, and thus retain some control.
	(c) Get away if possible.	(c) In order not to be trapped.
	(d) If you are trapped, try to use a piece of furniture as a shield.	(d) To protect yourself from injury.
	(e) Continue talking to the person.	(e) To convey that you feel in control of the situation, and to encourage the person to take a realistic view.
9. You are being approached by a person holding a sharp object.	9. (a) Shout loudly for help.	9. (a) To surprise your assailant.
	(b) Remain facing the person while backing away.	(b) So that you cannot be attacked from behind, and thus retain some control
	(c) Get away if possible	(c) In order not to be trapped.
	(d) If you are trapped, pick up some clothing or other material: for example, a cushion or towel.	(d) To protect yourself from injury by smothering the weapon if you are attacked.
	(e) Continue talking to the person.	(e) To convey that you feel in control of the situation, and to encourage the person to take a realistic view.

Problem	Action	Rationale
10. You are being approached by a person holding a firearm or explosive device.	10. (a) Do as the person says.	10. (a) In order not to put yourself or others at risk.
	(b) Avoid provoking the person.	(b) In order not to put yourself or others at risk.
11. A person armed with a weapon leaves the premises	11. Call the police, using 999.	11. To ensure that you hand over responsibility to them.
12. You are physically attacked while out in the community.	12. (a) Keep shouting and yelling.	12. It is essential to attract attention and to convince bystanders that you need help, and also to convince your attacker that he or she is likely to be caught if he or she persists.
	(b) Run to the nearest occupied building as soon as you can.	
	(c) Do not hesitate to defend yourself, for example by kicking, gouging, scratching, biting, and using keys or similar things as weapons.	
	(d) Try to impair your attacker's ability to see: for example, by rubbing mud in his or her eyes.	

Do's and Don'ts of home visiting

DO	DON'T
Dress inconspicuously.	Advertise your profession with car stickers and similar items which could be an invitation to drug-seekers.
Use a sports bag instead or a 'doctor's' bag.	Carry unnecessary equipment or drugs.
Use a car alarm which is linked to the boot as well as to the bonnet.	Leave any articles whatsoever inside the car when it is parked.
Always leave a schedule of your planned route and timetable before you go out.	Use an unreliable car.
Know your practice patch.	Wander about looking lost, or loiter if you are uncertain where you are.
Before a visit, familiarize yourself with your patients' notes and family history.	Rely on second- or third-hand reports.
Arrange a rendezvous with a relative of the patient if you feel uncertain of the area.	Accept guidance from strangers.
Ask to go with a colleague such as a community psychiatric nurse.	Be ashamed to ask for support.
Ask for a police escort if necessary.	Rely on a personal alarm. Who would hear it, and who would know what it was?
Take the dog.	Hang on to your bag if threatened.
Park your car nearby, especially when it is dark.	Leave it where it could be vandalized or where you could be ambushed.
On arrival try to memorize access and exit routes.	Leave yourself with a complicated route back to your car.
Keep fit, so that you are alert and can run if necessary.	Rely on learning karate.
Use stairs instead of the lift.	Hesitate to change your route if you think you are being followed.

DO	DON'T
Look out for likely houses or flats where you could seek help in an emergency.	Hesitate to lie about being expected home at a specific time.

Do's and don'ts in dealing with violence in long-stay institutions and between patients

DO	DON'T
Obtain practical training in 'breakaway' techniques.	Rely on theoretical knowledge.
Acknowledge that violent incidents will occur.	Assume that, with the best prevention, violence will never occur.
Develop a policy which works for your institution.	Rely on national guidelines.
Call for expert help to deal with fighting.	Intervene physically between antagonists without assistance.
Involve colleagues who know the patient(s) well.	Underestimate the value of the the presence of someone whom the antagonists know and trust.
Note and act on the mood-changes which often precede violence.	Wait until physical violence has erupted before intervening.
Agree with colleagues who will take charge of a situation BEFORE intervention.	Allow conflict between colleagues in the management of violent patients.

Do's and Don'ts when dealing with violent elderly people

DO	DON'T
Be aware that large numbers of staff can appear threatening to the elderly.	Force patients to fit in with your routine.
Be aware that violence in elderly people may be unpredictable.	Stereotype patients.
Identify calming influences for particular patients (eg photographs of young children or babies; a walk through the hospital grounds or a visit to the chapel).	Force attention on a patient who is hostile towards you.
Establish rapport prior to each intervention: violence often erupts when unprepared patients are suddenly required to comply with an instruction.	Expect elderly patients to understand that informal and casual clothes can be worn by qualified staff.

DO

Demonstrate non-possessive warmth and positive regard.

Involve chaplains, because the opportunity to pray or share the sign of the cross can be calming.

Managing aggressive animals in the home

Pet dogs are a part of many households. They are protective and territorial, and can perceive raised tensions in the home for example at times of illness or domestic crisis. An unknown visitor may be perceived as an intruder even by well-trained animals, though its owners may make light of the obvious signs of an aggressive reaction, for example growling, raised hackles, bared teeth. Always ask for dogs to be confined in another room before you enter the house.

Other problems which contribute to the development of violent incidents

Problem	Probable causes	Suggested actions
1. A patient or relative becomes agitated and distressed.	1. (a) They are in pain.	1. (a) Reassess and deal with the cause of the pain if necessary.
	(b) They are frightened	(b) Reassess and give information and guidance.
	(c) They are overwhelmed by their surroundings (for example, a noisy or crowded room).	(c) Remove sources of noise if possible. Move the person to a quieter place if possible.
	(d) They are uneasy about the area in which they find themselves or are being kept waiting.	(d) Ensure that patients and relatives can make telephone calls, use the lavatory, and obtain refreshments without fear of losing their place in any queue.

Problem	Probable causes	Suggested actions
1. A patient or relative becomes agitated and distressed. *(cont'd)*		(e) Set, maintain, and monitor standards for departmental activities, such as patients' waiting-times.
2. A member of staff is abrupt with a patient or relative.	2. He or she is inexperienced; or under stress; or dislikes some kinds of people.	2. (a) Maintain a system of supervision and appraisal for staff which ensures that less experienced staff work under supervision at first.
		(b) Use meetings to keep an eye on stress levels among staff, and relocate them to less stressful areas when possible.
		(c) Be aware of colleagues' strengths and weaknesses, and do not hesitate to offer help.
		(d) Always be prepared to ask for help yourself.
3. A person appears incoherent and cannot give a clear account of him- or herself.	3. (a) Intoxication	3. Ensure that patients are assessed by experienced staff.
	(b) Sensory impairment	Liaise with psychiatrically trained staff who can do a mental state assessment.
	(c) Acute psychosis	Maintain departmental procedures for managing intoxicated clients.
	(d) Cultural factors (for example, language difficulties)	Ensure that such patients are in a safe location, with adequate supervision if necessary.

Problem

3. A person appears incoherent and cannot give a clear account of him- or herself. (*cont'd*)

Probable causes

(e) Cerebral disorder (for instance secondary to trauma)

(f) Acute confusional state (for instance, secondary to infection or poisoning)

(g) Drug withdrawal

(h) Learning difficulties

Action

1. Identify risk patients: for example in homes where there is domestic violence; those known to have used violence in a health-care setting previously.

2. Ensure good lines of communication within the practice, whether by formal team meetings or daily casual contact.

3. Recognize the causes of complaint by patients – for example prolonged waiting-time without explanation, queues for registration, other delays in the service.

4. Recognize clinical issues that may cause conflict, and agree on a practice policy – for example, on the prescribing of tranquillizers or opiates for addicts, or on issuing sick notes.

5. Ensure that there is a system for making joint visits to difficult homes.

6. Make sure your complaints mechanism is readily accessible for patients and that any complaints are dealt with quickly and effectively.

Rationale

1. So that staff can be alerted. Nurses may choose to visit in pairs; doctors may choose to see a patient only with a colleague.

2. So that patterns of difficult behaviour can come to light early and be discussed from all points of view.

3. To reduce stress and frustration among patients and staff.

4. Setting clear limits by means of agreed practice policies may reduce uncertainty and stress for medical and nursing staff – and makes it easier to say no.

5. Staff may be reluctant to admit that they are concerned about their personal safety.

6. To reduce frustration and resentment and improve the quality of your service.

Action

Rationale

7. Use an Incident Book to record all episodes of aggressive behaviour.

7. To preserve details of episodes for later use. To enable you to seek appropriate resources such as extra staff or improvements to premises via the police, the FHSA, or the health authority.

8. Agree on guidelines for home visits in your area.

8. Helps staff new to the area. Supports staff faced with a threatening situation.

9. Strive to maintain a high-quality service in your practice – agree on basic standards, for example the maximum time to wait for a routine appointment or a repeat prescription.

9. To minimize complaints of all kinds.

10. Agree a practice policy on removal of patients after an aggressive incident.

10. To make all staff feel valued and to maintain morale, and so that patients understand that certain types of behaviour are unacceptable.

11. Stop routine work after an upsetting incident for an immediate debriefing period for all staff concerned.

11. To help express and anticipate the difficult and confused feelings that many victims experience.

12. Be prepared to allow staff home after an incident.

12. Some people prefer to express distress in private, and may, in any case, just need a rest.

13. Any member of staff who has felt sufficiently threatened to set off an alarm should be given the opportunity to be escorted home or given alternative work for that day.

13. Cumulative effects of apparently trivial incidents can build up stress levels.

14. Never minimize another person's distress. Always ask 'How do you feel?' (Never 'You're all right, aren't you?').

15. Check up on your colleagues in the days after an incident.

15. Recognizing these painful emotions early can help prevent prolonged psychological morbidity and avoidance behaviour later.

Action	Rationale
16. Insist on police involvement after any assault.	16. To support staff, and to demonstrate that violent behaviour will not be tolerated. Nearly all police authorities now liaise with Victim Support Schemes.
17. Advise staff to make a Criminal Injuries Compensation Claim after any injury.	17. To support staff.

Emergency tranquillization

If medical treatment is thought to be necessary for assaultive behaviour, it is often in the form of rapid neuroleptization: that is, oral or parenteral administration of neuroleptic medication with the aim of reducing symptomatic behaviour without excessive sedation. Although the actions of chlorpromazine and haloperidol have been shown to be equally rapid and effective, chlorpromazine can cause severe orthostatic hypotension when given parenterally. It is essential that the patient's blood pressure is measured as soon as possible after the administration of the drug, and it is helpful if the patient lies semi-prone for thirty minutes or so after the injection. In a crisis, where emergency tranquillization is unavoidable:

- Restrain your patients by holding their clothing, rather than their limbs.
- If the limbs are restrained they should be held at the large joints, to prevent fractures and other injuries.
- Do not press on the neck or chest.
- Tying the shoelaces together may help restrain the patient's legs.
- Alternatively, removing the shoes may prevent injuries caused by kicking.

Adequate doses of drugs must be given intramuscularly. The lateral thigh may be most accessible; and it may be necessary to inject through clothing. Doctors are advised to keep within the British National Formulary dose limits and to follow the recommendations of the Royal College of Psychiatrists until more is known about the complications of administering neuroleptic medication in high dosage.

After tranquillization, the patient's airway must be carefully monitored, and an airway must be inserted if there is any sign of respiratory obstruction. The patient is nursed having been placed, if possible, in the recovery position. Suction, and a bag and mask to assist ventilation must be available.

Guidelines for action after a violent incident

The incident must always be reported to the police. The staff chiefly
involved in the incident, especially from the beginning, must write
an account of what happened. This is useful in itself as evidence
if needed later, since a contemporary record is acceptable in court;
and it also allows staff to do some mental processing of the events
for themselves, to get some perspective, and perhaps to reassure
themselves that they took an acceptable course of action. This account
is sent as a report to the immediate supervisor of the staff involved,
who is responsible for discussing it with the senior manager, head
of department, or senior partner as appropriate. The staff member
should go to the Occupational Health Department for injuries to be
checked (no matter how apparently superficial) and to be recorded,
and to establish contact in case specialist counselling is needed at
a later date. It is advisable to ask for support from a professional
organization or one of the medico-legal protection societies, which
have, for example, undertaken to give legal advice and support to
doctors in this context (see Appendix I for addresses and telephone
numbers). Outside sources of support ranging from a local church to
a women's support group may be available.

Critical incident debriefing

In the growing field of post-traumatic stress disorder it has become
clear that helpers, including fire-fighters, police, nurses, teachers,
and dog-handlers may develop stress reactions following relatively
minor events, as well as disasters. Stress reactions are common
sequelae of violent attacks (see Chapter 1). These reactions, which can
emerge weeks and months after an event, may be diminished by the
use of the psychological intervention of debriefing following a critical
occurrence, 'critical occurrence' meaning here an event which produced in the person who experienced it a feeling of threat of harm.

The goals of the process are to assure the person that his or her
reaction is normal, and that the cohesiveness of the health-care team
is unaffected by the incident; to anticipate feelings and thoughts
which are likely to occur as time goes by; to reduce tension; and
to provide immediate and continuing support.

The process happens in three stages. First is the informal getting-
together of the work team, usually over tea or coffee (but not alcohol)
immediately after the event. Even if only one person was involved,
the team has a responsibility to drop its other work and attend this
group meeting, which may be led by someone senior in the practice
or hospital, though this should preferably be a member of staff who

has received training in stress-management. The group refrains from probing, hilarity, criticism, and requests for detailed descriptions of events, accepting that people may be unable or unwilling to go into what might have been a humiliating and terrifying experience. The second stage should begin one or two days after the event, again with the same people who attended the initial group. This second meeting is more formal, and is conducted in privacy, with at least two hours made available for it, in order to allow time for the leader to deliver an introduction to the session and an explanation of its ground rules and aims; for members to re-live the event; for members to talk about their responses to the event; for members to express their feelings and reactions; for members to talk about things at home; for the leader to provide educative material on the kinds of effects to expect, and to suggest ways in which group members might support each other over the coming weeks; and finally for the leader to explain how people can obtain further help. The third stage is a follow-up group meeting, whose format and timing is decided during the second stage.

FURTHER READING

Braithwaite, R. (1992). Violence—understanding, intervention and prevention. Radcliffe Professional Press, Oxford.

Cembrowicz, S. (1987). Assault on a GP. *British Medical Journal*, **294**, 616–18.

Cembrowicz, S.P. and Shepherd, J.P. (1992). Violence in the Accident and Emergency Department. *Medicine, Science, and the Law*, **32**, 118–21.

Crate, R. (1986). Social workers and violent clients: management response. *Social Work Today*, **10**, 14–15.

Emson, H.E. (1986). Violence and the doctor: 'ethics'. *Medicine, Science, and the Law*, **26** (3), 218–25.

Harris, A. (1989). Violence in General Practice. *British Medical Journal*, **298**, 63–4.

Health and Safety Executive (1987). *Violence to staff in the Health Service*. HMSO, London.

Lanza, M.L. (1985). How nurses react to assault. *Journal of Psychosocial Nursing and Mental Health Services*, **23** (6), 6–11.

Mitchell, J. (1983). When disaster strikes: the Critical Incident Stress Debriefing process. *Journal of Emergency Medical Services*, **8** (1), 36–9.

Whalen, J., Zimmerman, D.H., and Whalen, M.R. (1988). When words fail: a single-case analysis. *Social Problems*, **35** (4), 335–62.

3 Alcohol, other drugs, and violence

Duncan Raistrick

MORE THAN CAUSE AND EFFECT

At a nurse-training event a straw poll comparing the views of nurses working in an Accident and Emergency Department with nurses working in an Addiction Unit revealed interesting differences of perception regarding the relationship between violence and substance-use. Nurses were asked to think of a recent violent incident where alcohol or other drugs were also involved: the Accident and Emergency staff emphasized the role of alcohol in causing violent incidents, while the Addiction Unit staff saw the problem as having much to do with particular kinds of people harbouring a propensity for violence. Neither group questioned the implied association between violence and substance-use. Common sense and common experience seemed to underpin this association.

The question was important in demonstrating that the attribution of cause was less well informed and less to do with the violent incident than it was to do with making sense, *post hoc*, of each nurse's experience in practice and professional life. For the addiction nurses violent incidents were an unusual occurrence, and they felt comfortable suggesting that the individuals involved were really the province of the penal system rather than the treatment agency. It might be difficult to sustain professional self-esteem working with people who choose to use psychoactive substances, if the substances they used were, of themselves, expected to cause violence. For the accident and emergency nurses the opposite was true; violent incidents were more usual, and so, in order to make sense of caring for people in this kind of atmosphere, and sustain professional self-esteem, the problems were attributed to an external agent, in this case alcohol.

This anecdote illustrates the complexities of analysing commonly accepted associations, and especially so when dealing with behaviour such as violence and substance-misuse, where professional carers may themselves feel in double danger of acquiring some of the stigmatization or negative attitudes often directed at this behaviour. The natural and healthy response of the carers is to distort events in order to maintain their own integrity: in short to use defence mechanisms to account for their particular role. The straw poll illustrates a further problem which is inherent to survey or epidemiological research. The accident and emergency nurses reported only violent incidents involving alcohol, whereas the addiction nurses thought amphetamine equally a problem; in other words the population sampled and the rigour of that sampling will often be the major determinant of findings. These problems are well understood, and yet a trap for the unwary or uncritical observer.

THE FAMILY SETTING

In North America, the family as a source of learning that violence is an acceptable and normal part of a relationship has been identified: 50–90 per cent of violent incidents in the home occur while at least one family member is intoxicated, and about two-thirds of the cases involve alcohol, while one-third involve other drugs. What constitutes violence in the home has generally been defined in subjective terms of what is unacceptable to the recipient, rather than in terms of categorizing the behaviour. So, unacceptable aggression may be anything from pushing or slapping through to forced sex or assaults with weapons.

Support for a link between child-abuse, physical or sexual, and substance-misuse being transmitted in families is claimed from studies of young offenders. Among these young people there are high prevalence rates for misuse of illicit drugs and a consistent positive association with a range of childhood abuse, accounting directly for as much as 30 per cent of illicit drug use.

Disturbances of child development are difficult to rectify later in life, and especially so where there is dependence on alcohol or other drugs. It follows that it may be useful for carers to develop skills of remedial work with children in families where violence and substance misuse coexist. It has been argued that intoxication serves to excuse violent behaviour with the aim of maintaining family integrity: this is another example of the user, retrospectively, making sense of an unwanted behaviour; but, in common with most defence mechanisms, understanding is insufficient to inform action. So what protective interventions are available to the carer? Two general principles are useful: first, the less the disruption to family life the greater the chance of survival; and, second, the less the violence and substance misuse, the greater the chance of survival.

The first principle can be supported in different ways depending on how much family cohesion remains. At one extreme the task may simply involve securing stricter adherence to family routines such as meal-times, taking the children to school, quality time with parents, and regular bedtimes; at the other extreme remedial work may have more to do with practical, self-preservation ploys for the children, such as having a key to get in and out of the house, knowing who and how to telephone for help, and having a safe place to go.

The second principle may be difficult to support. The violent behaviour and substance-misuse behaviour should be tackled separately, possibly involving specialist help. The more unwanted behaviour there is in a household then the more coping strategies have to be used by partners and, to some extent, children; clearly a point may be reached where these coping strategies are failing or become exhausted altogether. So, alongside efforts to treat the unwanted behaviours directly, it may also be useful to teach partners coping skills: the general principle will be selectivity, and judiciously choosing to attack or ignore substance-misuse behaviours while encouraging agreeable interpersonal contacts. This is best done by working individually with partners and listing their responses to episodes of intoxication: having done this it is usually easy for partners to see which of their coping behaviours are likely to exacerbate substance-misuse and possibly aggression, and which will achieve the opposite and desired effect.

THE CULTURAL SETTING

Most violence associated with substance-misuse is thought to occur in the domestic setting, and therefore has implications for the transmission of both behaviours to new generations. This mechanism does not explain all the associations between crime, violence in particular, and substance-misuse; much debate has revolved around the question 'does drug misuse lead to crime or does crime lead to drug misuse?' There seems to be agreement that intoxication, rather than regular use, is behind much substance-related violence. At a very crude level of analysis it can be said that the criminal career, not necessarily violent, antedates the substance-misuse career about as often as the opposite is true. There is a strong association between progression of the substance-misuse career from licit to soft drugs, soft to hard drugs, and hard drugs to injecting drugs, and criminal activity of all kinds. Violence, including gang fights, assault, and armed robbery, has been reported as happening, on average, from 5 days a year for licit users to 36 days a year for injectors, though variations were quite marked within each group: violence may be related not only to the severity of drug-taking but also friends' drug-taking and to the extent of previous criminal history. The overview is of a teenage group where delinquent behaviour, including violence, vandalism, and experimentation with alcohol, solvents, cannabis, and to a lesser extent hard drugs, covary; each element nudges the other on a stage further (see Chapter 9).

Why do some adolescents grow out of this phase and others not? A lack of conventional social support and associating with friends that have criminal or drug-using backgrounds have also been shown to be important factors in the process of pushing an individual towards a life-style which embraces both crime and substance-misuse, the one feeding the other. Not all illegal drug-use involves violence, and not all legal use is peaceful. The difference is that the repertoire of violent behaviour grows with the progression from soft, legal to hard, illegal substance-use. Unfortunately these findings open up few easy opportunities for intervention, suggesting a need for fairly intensive individualized programmes.

THE VIOLENCE-FORMING POTENTIAL OF PSYCHOACTIVE SUBSTANCES

Intoxication, Tolerance, and Withdrawal

The previous section established an association between substance-misuse and violence, leaving open the question of how much the drug itself might contribute to that association. Some drugs are thought of in the public's mind as more likely to cause violent episodes than others: alcohol and cocaine might be taken as examples. However, as was discussed earlier, common beliefs may well be coloured by the prevalence of alcohol use, so that its connection with violence may prove, on close examination, a spurious one, whereas the connection between violence and cocaine use is found to be more solid. What then are the pharmacological effects of a drug that are likely to contribute to a violent episode?

An alteration of mental state to impair judgement, to release inhibitions, to confuse, to increase confidence, to increase activity, to induce paranoia, to distort perceptions, or to increase irritability might be expected to be one of the ingredients of a violent episode. There are many drugs that can cause such shifts in mental state either as an effect of intoxication or as a result of withdrawal from the drug. Intoxication refers to the pharmacological effect of taking a particular psychoactive substance, and should be distinguished from states such as being 'drunk' or 'stoned', which refer to the behaviour associated with taking a particular drug. Behaviour has much to do with circumstances and expectations: experienced observers have repeatedly been unable to predict intoxication, meaning plasma levels of a drug, from behaviour. The effect of a drug is more pronounced during the phase of increasing plasma levels when compared with that of a similar but decreasing plasma concentration.

As individuals use a drug on a regular basis over a period of time they become accustomed to its effect, and require a higher dose of the drug in order to achieve the same effect as on initial use. This phenomenon is referred to as tolerance, which is largely accounted for by a reduced sensitivity of the central nervous system. Learning to handle being intoxicated may contribute significantly to the overall tolerance; and, for some drugs, an increase in their rate of metabolism plays a part. Tolerance does not develop evenly for all the effects of a substance: for example tolerance to the sedative effect of alcohol is not matched by tolerance to its amnesic effect, and tolerance to the euphoriant effects of opiates is not matched by tolerance to their analgesic properties. In some situations tolerance may appear to decrease: for example, cannabis-smokers often improve their smoking technique so as to enhance, at least for a time, the drug effect, and drinkers often report a decline in tolerance, usually attributed to tissue damage, in the later stages of their drinking careers.

Withdrawal symptoms may occur in individuals who develop tolerance to a drug. In developing tolerance a kind of resistance or opposition to the effects of a drug is built up by changes in biochemical activity within the central nervous system: balance is created, so that the individual feels and functions more or less normally only when intoxicated with the drug or with a drug from a similar pharmacological group. If this drug is suddenly stopped then the biochemical shifts that were opposing and neutralizing the drug effect are released and manifest as withdrawal symptoms. Typically withdrawal symptoms are opposite in direction to the drug effect.

Method of use

The intensity of a desired drug effect and the propensity for the emergence of undesired effects, possibly with potential for aggression and violence, owes much to the particular preparation that is taken and how it is taken. In terms of both speed of onset and dose of drug delivered there is a hierarchy of methods of use which holds good for most substances: the least efficient is the oral route, which is both slow in terms of onset of effect and costly in terms of liver metabolism of the drug ingested; subcutaneous and intramuscular injection are probably on a par with snorting; intravenous injection and inhalation are the most effective routes. It is not just the route but also the preparation that is important: for example cocaine inhaled in the form known as CRACK will produce plasma levels five times those of a larger dose of snorted crystalline cocaine. Alcohol, which is normally taken as a drink, is most rapidly absorbed at a strength of 10–30 per cent, which coincides with the strength of drinks such as gin and tonic, sherry, and beer with a whisky chaser. In short, the choice of route of administration and of preparation of a substance may be calculated, usually through experience, to maximize the drug effect: the more profound the disturbance of mental state the more likely aggression and violence.

The severity of withdrawal symptoms depends upon the rate of fall of plasma levels of a substance, which, in turn depends upon the dose taken and the speed with which the substance is metabolized. A convenient measure is the half life of a substance, which is defined as the time taken to reduce the plasma level by 50 per cent. The practical implication is that, all other things being equal, a drug with a short half life such as morphine will require a dose every 6–8 hours in order to avoid withdrawal symptoms, whereas a different opioid drug, such as methadone, with a very long half life, will require only a once-daily dose. It follows that the drug with the shorter half life will have the greater potential for aggression and violence, in terms of both procurement needs and more rapid shifts to unpleasant mental states.

The setting

The effect of a drug may be modified and indeed wholly altered because of the circumstances in which it is taken. For example, being at a football match or a rock concert may, of itself, be more potent than a drug in heightening the level of arousal and excitement; equally, to be arrested by the police or to find oneself alone in an unfamiliar place may be a sobering experience. This capacity for shaping the effect of a drug is known as plasticity. Drugs that are said to be low in plasticity, such as heroin and amphetamine, have very predictable effects irrespective of the circumstances of their use, whereas highly plastic drugs, such as solvents and LSD, are dependent upon setting to define the drug experience. The most popular recreational drugs, alcohol and cannabis, fall between these two extremes. It is perhaps not surprising that highly plastic drugs fail to find favour for general recreational purposes. The practical implications will be apparent after considering drug-specific effects.

Dependence

Dependence is a psychological phenomenon which evades precise definition. It is to do with the extent to which thinking about substance-use and behaviour related to substance-use come to dominate a person's life. Dependence is best understood within the framework of social learning theory; it is not therefore seen as an all-or-none phenomenon, but rather as existing across a spectrum from low to high. The high-dependence individual is characterized by a preoccupation with a need to use a drug or drugs in order to modulate every emotion, every physical experience, every life-event: the perceived need for a drug will be more important than anything else happening at that time. The high-dependence individual will be a regular, probably daily, user, and will often have a fairly stereotyped pattern of use; intake may well be high also, but not necessarily so.

Dependence *per se* probably makes only a modest direct contribution to the association between violence and substance-misuse: the indirect implications are much greater. The cost, both financial and in time, of maintaining a high level of dependence on any substance is likely to be significant, and liable to end in conflict with a partner, workmates, or suppliers of drink or other drugs. Equally, a failure to maintain a substance-use pattern can provoke craving and interpersonal conflicts. So dependence will contribute to the likelihood of aggression and violence by indirect means, and to a lesser degree by associated episodes of intoxication.

CLASSIFICATION

The pharmacopoeia of psychoactive drugs, licit and illicit, is so extensive that any attempt at a typology will quickly reveal shortcomings. None the less, it will be useful for practical purposes to bring together those substances that have similar effects and, in the main, similar withdrawal states. Four groups have been selected:

  (i) stimulant drugs;
 (ii) depressant drugs;
(iii) opiate drugs; and
(iv) perception-altering drugs

These groups are not mutually exclusive: for example alcohol, a depressant, and LSD a perception-altering drug, both have an initial stimulant effect, while morphine, an opiate, has powerful depressant properties. None the less, there is an established utility to this classification.

Stimulant drugs

The most powerful compounds in this group are cocaine and amphetamine; less potent compounds include caffeine, nicotine, and a variety of sympathomimetics, such as pseudoephedrine, used in such proprietary preparations as nasal decongestants. Typically the effect of taking cocaine or amphetamine is a feeling of confidence and general well-being: thoughts are sharper and come more quickly, speech is quickened, and there is a general overactivity. Intoxicated people are usually witty and infectious fun to be with; however, if crossed or interupted they may become irritable and aggressive. Stimulants remove the need for sleep, reduce the appetite, and heighten sexual drive.

As the dose of stimulant increases to toxic levels so the picture changes to one of extreme agitation, persecutory ideas, visual hallucinations, and confusion, and physical abnormalities including hypertension, seizures, and eventually coma. The early stages can be controlled using minor tranquillizers, and beta-blockers within a supportive environment. Both intoxication and overdose with stimulant drugs may be mistaken for a hypomanic illness.

Intoxication and overdose with stimulant drugs both have a potential for violence. Overactive people are more likely to come into contact with others: conflict is likely as they try and take other people along with their latest good ideas, which may include sexual propositions. Add to this picture feelings of great physical strength and suspicious or frankly deluded thinking, and violence becomes almost inevitable. Interestingly, regular users of stimulants are familiar with the experience of paranoid thoughts, and often retain sufficient insight to remove themselves from the company of others until their thoughts return to normal, which usually happens without recourse to specific treatment over 3–10 days.

The withdrawal, or come down, from cocaine and amphetamine is characterized by a depression of mood, which may be so profound as to require short-term hospitalization. Exhaustion is matched by an excess of sleep, but disturbed by troublesome and morbid nightmares. In short, any aggression at this stage is likely to be turned inwards.

Ecstasy is often included as a stimulant drug but can be seen as belonging to a separate group if preferred. Ecstasy and similar drugs combine amphetamine and LSD effects. Tolerance to the perception-altering properties happens quite quickly but the emotional bonding, which is seen to be the hallmark feature of the drug, persists; much of this can be attributed to the setting, usually a 'rave'.

Biographical snapshot

Around the turn of the century medical practitioners were more likely than members of any other profession to be addicted to cocaine. Sigmund Freud was perhaps the most famous of these physicians. After about 1892 biographers write of a change in Freud's personality characterized by marked swings of mood, an outpouring of work, indiscriminately placing sex at the centre of his analytical theories, and an intolerance, even a hatred, for old friends and colleagues, most notably Joseph Breuer. Freud's potential for violence was in fact contained, not least because he enjoyed the reputation of a genius rather than of a psychotic. Interestingly, Freud failed to connect the 'murderous and sadistic lusts' of his own dreams with cocaine use, preferring an analytical interpretation. So the picture with cocaine is of a drug with little respect for setting or character: stimulants induce a sense of arousal and power coupled with paranoia.

Depressant drugs

Numerically this is the largest group of psychoactive substances, and includes alcohol, minor tranquillizers, barbiturates, hypnotics, and other sedatives. It is probably useful to include cannabis within this group, since it is normally smoked, in the UK at least, as a relaxant. If preferred cannabis can, however, be set in a group of its own. It is usually held that drugs with a relatively non-specific mode of action, such as alcohol and barbiturates, impair higher cortical control centres in the brain, thereby disinhibiting the expression of emotions, thoughts, and behaviours normally not seen. The intoxicated person becomes more talkative, and may feel highly confident or even omnipotent, but in reality is less able to process information and is operating with impaired judgement. Setting aside any latent aggression or antisocial personality characteristics, there is scope here for any normal, well-adjusted person to misinterpret interactions or events, thereby increasing the potential for a violent outcome. The benzodiazepine tranquillizers, such as diazepam (Valium) and lorazepam (Ativan) have a specific effect on neurotransmitters, and the mode of action of cannabis is unknown: for practical purposes, however, the consequences of intoxication with it are very similar to those found with other depressants.

In contrast to the stimulant drugs, the risk of violence diminishes as the dose of depressant increases; and as matters progress the

capacity for co-ordinated movement is lost, and ultimately coma
supervenes. There is no specific treatment for depressant overdose.
Care should be taken to protect against inhalation of vomit, especially
when alcohol has been consumed; and hospitalization may be
necessary when a cocktail of depressants has been taken or when
consciousness is difficult to maintain. Cannabis is again an anomaly
here, in that overdose is characterized by a state of anxiety and fear
which may progress into a paranoid and confused state akin to that
described for stimulants, but without the overactivity: talking down
is usually sufficient.

There are three distinct phases of depressant withdrawal. First,
and by far the most common, is the tremulous state, which is
characterized by shakiness of hands, tremulousness of the face and
whole body, tachycardia, anxiety, and dysphoria; in more severe
cases there may be fleeting hallucinations and illusory distortions of
the immediate environment. In short, the potential for violence stems
from a state of over-arousal. These symptoms emerge within 6–8
hours of stopping drinking. A similar tremulousness and irritability
may be seen after heavy cannabis smoking.

For alcohol, benzodiazepines, and barbiturates a second phase
of withdrawal may be manifest as seizures; for alcohol these usually occur 24–36 hours after stopping drinking. A third and still
later phase, usually 72 hours after stopping drinking, is delirium: the delirium is often characterized by very frightening visual
hallucinations, often brightly coloured images of menacing animals such as rats, snakes, and spiders, and is often associated
with paranoid ideas. There is a marked increase in the likelihood
of violence, which will be directed against the hallucinations or
delusions.

Biographical snapshot

In Western countries alcohol is the most widely used legal recreational drug, and is often used by lovers and friends in social settings.
Caitlin Thomas, in her biography of Dylan Thomas, describes him
as a passive man, indeed a pacifist; and yet their drinking sessions
together were frequently scenes of argument, though it seems not
physical violence. Writing of one row she says, 'I can't remember
how it started but . . . everywhere was covered in green toothpaste
. . . neither of us could remember what happened . . . probably
something to do with women'. She describes herself as ashamed
of a visit to America because of 'all that drinking and fighting
(verbal)', and yet excuses her husband on the grounds of his
being a poet! In short, the picture is one of family and marital

neglect related to drinking, interspersed with frequent arguments while intoxicated.

Opiates

Opiates include all those substances that have a morphine-like effect. Most commonly misused are diamorphine (heroin), morphine, methadone (Physeptone), dihydrocodeine (DF118), codeine, and buprenorphine (Temgesic). The opiates work through specific receptors within the brain and receptors associated with smooth muscle. The most striking effect is a state of euphoria, or feeling on 'cloud nine', but in a dreamy sort of way and one that is detached from the immediate surroundings. An overdose of opiates simply enhances this state, but will cause respiratory depression and possibly death from respiratory failure. The effects of opiates can be reversed with naloxone (Narcan). Violence is an unusual companion of the opiate effect.

Withdrawal from opiates may be quite trivial, rather like a cold: a runny nose and eyes, and hot and cold sweats, but progressing in more severe withdrawal to muscle cramps, and sometimes to spasms, vomiting, and diarrhoea, with some degree of agitation. Because opiates work at specific receptors the effect of giving more opiate is completely and quickly to reverse the withdrawal state. It is in the pursuit of more opiates to avoid or relieve withdrawal that there is risk of violence. One of the arguments for long-term prescribing of methadone is that, because methadone has a very long half-life, repeated withdrawals, the associated craving for more opiates, and the potential for violence are reduced.

Biographical snapshot

It is generally the case that naturally occurring substances are moderate in their effects, and it is purified forms that take on the mantle of dangerousness. So it is with opiates. None the less, Thomas De Quincey in *Confessions of an English opium eater* captures very vividly the essence of opiate use (opium being the 'milk' of opium poppy). Contrasting opium with alcohol, he writes 'the man who is inebriated is in a condition which calls up into supremacy the merely human, too often the brutal, part of his nature: but the opium-eater feels that the diviner part of his nature is paramount; that is the moral attentions are in a state of cloudless serenity'. Later on he declares 'opium had long ceased . . . spells of pleasure; it was solely by the tortures connected with the attempt to abjure it, that it kept its hold', giving an insight that the opiate effect, rather than withdrawal, is central to opiate addiction.

Perception-altering drugs

Perception-altering drugs are something of a mixed bag, which contains solvents, butane gas and other volatile substances, LSD, and magic mushrooms. In contrast to the previous drug categories described, where the drug effect is essentially an extension of normal experience, the perception-altering drugs have the capacity to cause experiences outside the usual perceptual experience of reality, or, in other words, transient psychotic states. Volatile substances in particular endow the user with the capacity to experience illusory images which may amuse, but which may bring fear, aggression, or morbid thoughts. Volatile substances commonly act as depressants, and so a picture similar to alcohol intoxication may be superimposed on the illusory state; at higher doses there may also be hallucinations. LSD is an extremely potent drug which induces colourful and vibrant visual hallucinations. It is also a highly plastic drug, and so the content of the hallucinations may vary from being fun to being threatening and fear-provoking: the potential for violence varies accordingly. The psychosis of intoxication is best dealt with by reassurance from a trusted person who will encourage concentration to be focused on real verbal or visual stimuli; hypnotics may be useful, and major tranquillizers should be used if the psychosis persists beyond a few days. Some volatile substances have a withdrawal state similar to the tremulousness of depressants. There is no equivalent for LSD, even though experienced users become tolerant to doses 10–20 times those sufficient for naive users.

Biographical snapshot

Because LSD is such a highly plastic drug its potential for causing violence is largely determined by the circumstances of its use; and so the link between LSD and violence may be difficult to prove. The multiple murders committed by Charles Manson and his followers have, however, been linked to LSD. It may well be that Manson's underlying delusional symptoms were born out of a schizophrenic illness but enriched by his daily use of 'acid'. LSD may have had an additional and even more important role in altering the mental state of his followers so that they became more receptive and committed to an ideology embracing the need for ritual killing. In short, the picture is of a drug with so-called 'mind-expanding' properties, often appealing to those interested in 'alternative' life-styles, but with an effect conditioned by the setting in which it is taken.

PERSONAL FACTORS

Personality

The previous section has argued that the pharmacological effects of different drugs and the withdrawal symptoms associated with some substance-use are, of themselves, likely to increase the risk of violence. Equally some individuals will be more susceptible to the pharmacological processes than others. Students are often taken as the subjects for research in the addiction field, since they tend to use rather more alcohol and other drugs than the general population: as a group they are also more privileged in terms of educational achievement and future prospects. Although it might be expected that there would be low levels of violence among this group, the opposite has been found: in one study 20 per cent of males and 6 per cent of females admitted to damaging property after drinking, and 4 per cent of males and 5 per cent of females admitted to involvement in an assault. Some 20 per cent of males and 10 per cent of females had been assaulted by another college member who had been drinking. Assaults and vandalism have been associated with heavier drinking patterns; but there is no way of knowing whether alcohol was a causal agent or whether those people who drank heavily were also more aggressive. However, with such large numbers of students reporting involvement in assaults or vandalism it is tempting to believe that, given the combination of the right circumstances and intoxication, any individual has the potential for violence.

It has been seen, however, that crime in general is a function of antisocial personality. Drinking or drug use probably potentiates antisocial behaviour, and vice versa, though some would go so far as to say that without adverse personality characteristics drinkers or drug users are no more likely than anyone else to be violent. While it may be possible to support this view by studying the co-variance of the disorders antisocial personality and substance-misuse, the thesis depends upon acceptance of antisocial personality as a discrete condition. In reality definitions of antisocial personality are circular, and the characteristic is best understood as existing as a continuum. Equally, the extent of substance-use can be understood as existing as a continuum. The two continua are not entirely independent of each other, and interactions can be expected at all points.

A variant of the antisocial personality is the impulsive personality, meaning people who act without thinking and without awareness of the consequences: again the definition is somewhat circular. Impulsivity is not seen as a condition or disorder, but as a character trait that is distributed throughout the population. More impulsive individuals are more likely to be involved in a range of so-called impulsive behaviour, such as excessive drinking, drug use, gambling, bulimia, aggression, and self-harm.

A society that lives with and expects violence will be one where violence is generally more likely, but also one where it is more likely as a first-resort solution to problems. None the less, some kinds of violence have been associated with physiological factors. Taking homicide as the extreme of violence, where homicide is substance-related the offenders are more likely to have abnormal brain function. One study found that half the alcohol-abusers who had caused another's death had a degree of dementia, and/or withdrawal seizures, and/or alcoholic delirium. Equally the users of other drugs were likely to have a brain lesion or a history of psychotic episodes.

Victims

In the study of homicides referred to above, both the offender and victim were intoxicated except in a very small minority of cases. Where alcohol was misused the victim and offender were more intimate both in terms of their relationship and the method of killing: repeated stabbing, kicking, beating, and strangling were most common. Killings associated with illicit drug use are more likely to take place in public places and are more likely to be motivated by illicit drug trading than by passion. This probably reflects the fact that alcohol is the drug most commonly taken for social and recreational purposes.

The availability within a population of different substances and different weapons will determine the general level of their use, and this proposition also holds within subsections of the population. A North American study, for example, found that some 10 per cent of pregnant women were physically or sexually abused; the chances of being subject to violence increased up to 40 per cent, however, if the women drank heavily or took illicit drugs. At least one follow-up study of the victims of battery has found that of those who kill their batterers, the difference is with the men that batter rather than the women battered: the men killed were much more likely to be intoxicated on a daily basis and have a greater intake of both street and prescription drugs.

About 70 per cent of assault victims attending Accident and

Emergency Departments in Britain have taken alcohol in the six hours prior to assault: broadly speaking the victims have higher consumption levels and spend proportionately more of their income on alcohol than would be expected from the general population. In younger age-groups, however, drinking alone does not distinguish victims from other young males except where between seven and fifteen units of alcohol have been consumed, when injury is more likely. Consistent with this, there is a relationship between high binge consumption and severe injury in assault. Violence is often instigated by the eventual victim.

A rather different problem arises where individuals believe they have been assaulted, usually sexually, while under the influence of drugs: complaints of sexual assault, when assault could have happened, are well known in association with benzodiazepine sedation or anaesthesia. Equally benzodiazepines, alcohol, and other drugs have been given, usually to women, to facilitate rape and to fog the women's recollections of the sexual assault.

The concept of so-called 'date rape' once again brings substance misuse and violence out of the closet. It is no longer good enough to pretend that these behaviours are the monopoly of 'deviants' in the population; the goal is to change social attitudes and values more generally.

MEANING AND MANAGEMENT

Same violence – different reasons

The well-established association between violence and substance-misuse is seen to be crude when account is taken of violence as an end-point that can be reached by many routes. Take for example a serious assault causing actual bodily harm, and consider the possible reasons. First, an assault may be an act of enforcement. A drug dealer or liquor trader has a business to protect, and any weakness in collecting payment or defending a particular patch could quickly lead to the collapse of the business: this kind of violence may well occur as part of organized crime, and spill over into gang wars. A similar kind of problem may arise from disputes about the quality and quantity of the, usually illicit, drugs being dealt. 'Enforcement' violence is clearly a police matter.

Second, an assault may be to do with the effects of intoxication. In this case violence may be a way of communication for the inarticulate, an expression of anger for the introverted, or a consequence of misunderstanding for the person who has impaired judgement.

People tend to get intoxicated with people they know, and, in so far as this happens, then 'communication' violence will be directed at a friend, partner, or relative; in another sense the violence will be undirected and lack real purpose. It may be possible to deal with simple intoxication without involving the police: much depends upon the willingness of the individual to move to a safe place, which may be home, a hospital, or designated 'drying out' centre.

A third reason for an assault is mental illness as a result of intoxication or withdrawal. Mental illness in this context does not include personality problems, but rather refers to a state, albeit temporary, where there is a loss of contact with reality: in these states it becomes apparent that an individual's behaviour is actually a response to frightening hallucinations or delusional ideas that contain some element of threat. Drug-induced psychotic states are to be distinguished from functional psychosis by the presence of confusional and affective elements in the mental state. Individuals thought to be a danger can be detained under the Mental Health Act, even though the mental illness is substance-related. Many such psychotic states are ephemeral, lasting only a few hours or days. None the less, any case of delirium (meaning confusion, disorientation, or hallucinations, which are usually visual and secondary delusions), or any case of paranoid psychosis (meaning well-formed delusions or disorganized thought), where some threat is perceived, should be treated in a hospital setting, or at least under the direction of a clinician experienced in the field of mental illness and substance-use.

Checking out substance-misuse

Whatever the cause of violence, the behavioural management, from the viewpoint of health professionals, is initially the same: the objective will be to ensure the safety of staff, patients, and others present. The precise action will depend upon circumstances, and the general principles are discussed elsewhere in this book. It may or may not be obvious at the outset that a violent situation, potential or actual, is substance-related, and so it is useful for health care professionals to have a checklist in mind. Naturally the checklist will need the application of common sense to modify the approach in different settings.

Is the aggression substance-related?

In the majority of cases, it is self-evident that substance-use at least contributes to a situation: the individual will often be known, both sober and intoxicated; there will be a history from friends or relatives. In the absence of obvious signs it is still most likely that abnormal behaviour, particularly in young people, is substance-related; if appropriate, check pockets or handbags for drugs, enquire in a matter-of-fact, non-judgemental tone about possible use, and look for external signs such as injection marks, abnormal pupillary reactions, or indicator stains or marks on clothing. If possible a urine sample for toxicology screening and a blood sample for an alcohol level will be useful investigations: depending on the sensitivity of the assay, substances are likely to be detected in urine for 3–4 half lives after ingestion. For example, cocaine will very rarely be detected, except as its metabolite; whereas cannabis may be detected for more than one week after a single smoke.

Is the aggression caused by simple intoxication?

It may only be possible to make a preliminary judgement. The ideal solution is to place the person somewhere that they can 'sleep it off', 'come down', 'sober up': in other words environmental manipulation without prescribing medication is usually adequate. A 'carrot and stick' approach is worth practising: first apply the 'stick' in the form of overwhelming odds, discreetly available in the background; then apply the 'carrot' in the form of a personal approach which will be sympathetic, and concerned to resolve immediate problems. The intoxicated person may misunderstand conversation, leading to further aggression, and is likely to be amnesic for some parts of the discussion: it follows that the carer should give very clear and simple statements about what is going on, and not expect a therapeutic session at this point. The immediate task is to isolate the source of violence in a safe place where further assessment can be made. Any appointments, perhaps with a local addiction service, should be given in writing, with the sentiment that the carer is anxious that the patient or client should seek help.

Is the aggression caused by an abnormal mental state?

It is probable that containment of any aggression caused by psychosis will be symptom-rather than diagnosis based. However medication should, if possible, be withheld until after a psychiatric assessment. The important exception to this rule is Wernicke's encephalopathy, which is caused by thiamin deficiency associated with chronic alcoholism or carcinoma of the stomach, and which should be dealt with as an emergency, with the administration of intravenous thiamin. Drug-induced psychoses are frequently associated with confusion and disorientation: the essential action here is for a staff member to remain in constant contact as far as possible, to keep external stimuli to a minimum, and to give regular reality-orientation. The environment should be well lit, but with plain furnishings. The same principles apply where an individual is experiencing abnormal perceptions, particularly visual hallucinations, as part of delirium or intoxication with perception-altering drugs. Paranoid states either emerge from intoxication with drugs such as the stimulants or cannabis, or present as secondary symptoms as part of delirium, and in either event they require no specific treatment; chronic paranoid states, particularly when occurring in clear consciousness, should be treated as a functional psychosis.

Are there other problems to check out?

Having decided that someone is intoxicated, there is always a danger of becoming blind to the possibility of coexisting illness such as diabetes, chest infection, heart failure, head injury, or meningitis – all these are over-represented among people who misuse alcohol and other drugs. These conditions may themselves lead to aggression. In short, beware of intoxication masking other conditions which may require urgent attention. Equally, be aware of the possibility of future complications: check out the likelihood of a single-drug or a polydrug overdose, a history of seizures, delirium, or any other medical condition that would indicate hospital admission.

The attempt here has been to highlight some issues specific to substance-use and violence. Always these specific points are to be taken alongside general approaches to containing violence, and always to be applied with generous amounts of common sense, drawing upon any relevant disciplines and established knowledge concerned with treating the problems of addiction.

SUMMARY

Both substance-misuse and violence are behaviours that attract negative responses: professionals and patients alike distance themselves from any stigma by making sense of the behaviours *post hoc*. Both behaviours can be learned and transmitted in the family. The relationship between substance-misuse and violence is, however, complex: the more illicit and more deviant addictive behaviours are associated with more violence, but each potentiates the other.

Violence most commonly accompanies intoxication, but may also be associated with withdrawal symptoms and, usually in indirect ways, with high levels of dependence. The four major categories of psychoactive substances, namely stimulant drugs, depressant drugs, opiates, and perception-altering drugs can all cause, in some way or another, changes of mental state that increase the possibility of violence. Given the right mix of circumstances and drug effect most individuals have a potential for aggression or violence. Subgroups of the population with histories of physiological disturbance in brain function or organic brain syndromes are more prone to extremes of violence under the influence of psychoactive drugs.

The appropriate management of aggression depends upon an accurate assessment of its meaning. Health-care workers need to be clear about which situations demand a response from the police and which demand medical interventions. Health-care workers need to adapt general principles of managing violence to suit their particular work setting and professions.

FURTHER READING

Abram, K. M. (1989). The effect of co-occurring disorders on criminal careers: interaction of antisocial personality, alcoholism, and drug disorders. *International Journal of Law and Psychiatry*, **12**, 133–48.

Bennett, G. (1989). *Treating drug abusers*. Routledge, London.

Gorney, B. (1989). Domestic violence and chemical dependency: dual problems, dual interventions. *Journal of Psychoactive Drugs*, **21**, 229–38.

Hammersley, R. Forsyth, A., and Lavelle, T. (1990). The criminality of new drug users in Glasgow. *British Journal of Addiction*, **85**, 1538–94.

Lindqvist, P. (1991). Homicides committed by abusers of alcohol and illicit drugs. *British Journal of Addiction*, **86**, 321–6.

McGuire, P. and Fahy, T. (1991). Chronic paranoid psychosis after misuse of MDMA ('ecstasy'). *British Medical Journal*, **302**, 697.

Raistrick, D. R. and Davidson, R. (1985). *Alcoholism and drug addiction*. Churchill Livingstone, Edinburgh.

Shepherd, J. P. (1990). Alcohol and violence. *Lancet*, **336**, 1223–4.

Shepherd, J. Irish, M. Scully, C., and Leslie, I. (1989). Alcohol consumption among victims of violence and among comparable UK populations. *British Journal of Addiction*, **84**, 1045–51.

Smith, D. E. and Seymour, R. B. (1985). Dream becomes nightmare: adverse reactions to LSD. *Journal of Psychoactive Drugs*, **17**, 297–303.

Velleman, R. (1992). Intergenerational Effects—A review of environmentally oriented studies concerning the relationship between parental alcohol problems and family disharmony in the genesis of alcohol and other problems. II: The intergenerational effects of family disharmony. *The International Journal of the Addictions*, **27**, 367–89.

West, R., Drummond, C., and Eames, K. (1990). Alcohol consumption, problem drinking and antisocial behaviour in a sample of college students. *British Journal of Addiction*, **85**, 479–86.

4   Management of violent patients

Henrietta Bullard

Mentally disordered offenders account for a disturbing proportion of the remand and sentenced population in prison. A study of 2743 men admitted to a remand prison found that 9 per cent showed major symptoms of psychiatric illness and a further 8.6 per cent demonstrated symptoms of withdrawal from alcohol or other drugs. Of the men diagnosed as psychotic, 70 per cent suffered from schizophrenia. Not all these men were charged or convicted of offences involving violence; but 11 per cent of the homicides and 30 per cent of the arson offences were committed by men diagnosed as suffering from schizophrenia. The corresponding figures for depression were 2 per cent of homicides and no cases of arson.

The majority of psychiatric patients are disturbed but not aggressive. The word 'disturbed' carries different meanings for different people in a variety of situations. When used to describe a psychiatric patient, it generally implies that the patient's behaviour is disturbed. A patient who believes himself to be dead or one who claims to be the reincarnation of Moses will not be described as disturbed unless he behaves unconventionally. The word aggressive, on the other hand, is more specific; it implies verbal or physical threat or actual physical harm. Why are some psychiatric patients threatening and aggressive and others not? This is a complicated subject, and relates to a number of factors including the gender of patients, their pre-morbid personality, the type of mental disorder, and whether they are frightened, irritable, suspicious, excitable, angry, or a combination of all these.

Environmental factors are particularly important: most serious violence does not occur in psychiatric hospitals, where the patient is supervised and provided with structure and support. It is much more likely to occur in the patients' homes, where they are exposed to stress in their relationships with their families. A high proportion of patients who subsequently become violent have had admissions to psychiatric hospitals and been discharged to live in the community. The quality of care, whether in hospital or in the community, may have a profound effect on the potential for violence.

Mental disorder is defined in the Mental Health Act 1983 as meaning 'mental illness, arrested or incomplete development of mind (mental impairment), psychopathic disorder and any other disorder or disability of mind'. Mental illness is not defined in the Mental Health Act or in the International Classification of Mental Disorders of 1978, but by convention is used to include the psychotic, neurotic, and organic brain disorders.

Schizophrenia

Schizophrenia is a common and often damaging mental illness. The majority of patients in psychiatric hospitals, and now increasing numbers in the community, have schizophrenia. It affects nearly 1 per cent of the population, and its effects on the lives of sufferers and their relatives are profound. There is a slight preponderance of males, and the illness characteristically presents in late adolescence and early adult life. The onset of the illness may be abrupt or insidious. There is often a prodromal period when the young person becomes less sociable and fails to achieve his or her potential at school. They may 'drop out' and behave in an uncharacteristic manner: neglecting their appearance, and sometimes abusing illegal drugs. Some patients become interested in psychology, philosophy, and the paranormal. This period of the illness is followed by increasingly bizarre behaviour, associated with hallucinations, abnormal beliefs (delusions), and difficulty with language. Many patients experience paranoid delusions, which they hold with unshakeable conviction. These delusions cause great distress, and some patients feel persecuted and victimized all their lives. They may complain that their minds or bodies have been 'taken over', and that none of their thoughts are their own. One patient killed himself in prison after many years of believing that the Home Office were electronically spying on his brain. He wore a metal foil hat to prevent penetration of the 'rays'. This patient was not susceptible to rational argument, and had no insight into his illness. He was nevertheless suffering as a result of his delusions, and during a period of low mood killed himself. It is sometimes not appreciated that 10 per cent of patients with schizophrenia kill themselves. Suicide may be the result of intolerable and protracted paranoid delusions, or, tragically, can occur when patients develop insight into their illness and recognize the hopelessness of their situation.

One of the most serious consequences of schizophrenia is the gradual deterioration in the personality. Once lively and energetic young people with a zest for life become strange and withdrawn. They may have difficulty in caring for themselves and neglect their personal hygiene. As the illness progresses the more florid symptoms usually subside, and patients are left with a 'defect state'. This describes a state in which there is loss of drive and initiative, and patients may not even be able to get up in the morning without prompting. Our large psychiatric hospitals, which are now closing or have already closed, were home for thousands of schizophrenic patients who were thought to need asylum. The concept of asylum and institutional care is now an unfashionable one, and the current trend is for care in the community.

Treatment is available for patients with schizophrenia, and this is usually started in hospital. The phenothiazine drugs, for example chlorpromazine and the depot preparations of phenothiazines, do help most patients. These drugs are particularly effective in suppressing or alleviating the florid symptoms, including delusions and hallucinations, usually found in schizophrenia. Patients who do respond to treatment regain insight, and are often willing to continue medication when they leave hospital. This is known to be very important; and patients who relapse are often found to have discontinued medication before becoming ill. A proportion of patients remain psychotic and resistant to modern drugs. These patients cannot hope to live normal lives in the community.

Most patients with schizophrenia never show physical violence and never commit offences. Patients with schizophrenia tend to be withdrawn and non-assertive. However, a minority of patients do become verbally and physically aggressive, and it is important that for this minority the circumstances leading to violent episodes are understood and properly monitored. Many of the patients who commit serious offences of violence and require treatment in one of the three special hospitals (Broadmoor, Rampton, and Ashworth) have a history of previous psychiatric treatment associated with threats of violence or actual violence. The prediction of violence is fraught with difficulties, but doctors and other professionals must be alert to the possibility of dangerous behaviour. The risk will be higher if the patients have a history of assaults or have used weapons; if they have expressed an intention to harm or kill; if they have a named victim or victims; and if their illnesses have relapsed. Families are often at most risk, and, because of the homelessness associated with mental illness (schizophrenia in particular), the mentally ill are often cared for by elderly parents. The presence of a mentally ill son or daughter in the family home is stressful for everyone and, if patients harbour paranoid delusions about their families and are not receiving any psychiatric treatment they may, in response to their illnesses, erupt into violence. There is evidence that where family violence and schizophrenia are associated, the mother is most at risk.

Manic-depressive psychosis

The manic and the depressed patient both suffer from a disorder of mood, and both conditions may co-exist in the same patient at different times. Manic-depressive psychosis is the name given to an illness characterized by pathological fluctuations in mood. The manic patient is irritable, overactive, and disinhibited. He feels wonderful, and may describe grandiose delusions, perhaps believing himself to be a famous brain surgeon or related to royalty. He talks incessantly, and ideas come tumbling out: some make sense, some do not. Although manic patients are risks to themselves through spending their money recklessly, making unconsidered sexual liaisons, and by restless overactivity, they rarely inflict serious violence. Such patients are difficult to manage in the community, and urgently need hospital admission. Because of their exuberance in public places they are often picked up by the police. The police need to exercise considerable skill and judgement when handling a manic patient, who will probably not want to co-operate. The police are often subjected to assaults, usually punches and kicks, by manic patients, who may cause a considerable disturbance in a police station. A police cell is not a very appropriate place for someone who is mentally ill; but it usually has to do until the patient can be detained under the Mental Health Act and transferred to hospital.

The depressed patient suffers from a pathologically low mood, as a consequence of which he is unable to make rational judgements. His whole outlook on life is coloured by his depressive disorder which will also influence his behaviour. Suicidal ideas are common, and 15 per cent of depressed patients succeed in committing suicide at some time. There is a high risk of suicide in women who kill their children and in men who kill their wives. While depression is associated with homicide, this is always in the context of the family, while homicides committed by patients suffering from schizophrenia are more random. Depressed patients rarely, if ever, kill strangers.

Neurotic disorders

The neurotic disorders include anxiety states, obsessive compulsive disorders, and hysterical phenomena. Neuroses are life-long disabling conditions, but they do not involve the patient in loss of contact with reality. Neurotic patients know there is no substance to their anxiety, but continue to suffer as if there were. There is a condition called a 'dissociative state' or 'fugue state' which is commonly seen in neurotic patients who also have hysterical features. These patients react to stress by psychological denial. They no longer feel in contact with themselves or their problems, and during these periods of altered consciousness may behave bizarrely. It is very rare for patients to be violent while in a dissociative state, although less serious acquisitive offending may occur.

Personality disorders

People are not all the same, but most people conform to the basic rules of a civilized society. We do not kill unless seriously provoked or in self-defence; we do not rape or cause physical harm to others. If we do harm to or injure another person we feel guilt and remorse. There are some people who know the rules but do not or cannot comply with them. Aggressive psychopaths who are persistently assaultive probably have little or no control over aggressive impulses. They themselves may have been the victims of violence, and their reactions and behaviour have been modelled on those of their parents. They can be very dangerous, and particularly when under the influence of alcohol. They may however show genuine remorse, and not all psychopathic personalities have the cold, emotionless inner world that is usually ascribed to them.

The sexual psychopath, who is fortunately very rare, may only demonstrate his potential for violence in a sexual context. Abnormal sadistic sexual fantasies are private and hidden until they are acted out in a sexual assault. The sadistic sexual psychopath needs violence, in either fantasy or reality, to become sexually aroused to the point of ejaculation.

Inadequate-personality disorders are commonly associated with self-mutilation, para-suicide, and sometimes arson. Serious violence is uncommon unless in a domestic setting. Inadequate people are often dependent, and sensitive to loss or rejection. Men who kill their wives are usually both dependent and depressed. There may have been a deterioration in the relationship, possibly due to the wife's need for more freedom and autonomy. He may interpret his wife's interest outside the home as a criticism and rejection of himself. These feelings may then turn to rejection and anger. An insecure inadequate man may decompensate for his ability to cope with the stress of real or imagined loss, and, in a mood of depression mixed with anger and resentment, he loses control and kills his wife. He kills the person he loves the most, and on whom he depends.

Delusional jealousy is the term used to describe a syndrome where the patient becomes convinced his wife or girlfriend (usually wife) is unfaithful. He goes to extreme lengths to 'catch her out', and may examine her knickers for semen stains and go through her handbag for clues of infidelity. The underlying disorder is usually schizophrenia, and the outlook for recovery is poor.

Mental impairment

The mentally handicapped, whether or not the intellectual deficit is substantial, have difficulties in learning and acquiring sufficient skills to confront a complex world. The severely handicapped cannot live independently, but in some cases demonstrate unpredictable and violent behaviour. Their aggression is usually non-directional and unpredictable. Nursing staff need to have accepted procedures for controlling and restraining severely handicapped patients during aggressive outbursts. The minimum of force must be used, and every effort needs to be made to calm and relax the patient.

Mild degrees of mental handicap may be associated with minor sexual offending, and occasionally with more serious offences, including arson and sexual violence. The physical and sexual abuse of children may occur in families where both partners are intellectually impaired. Social deprivation, including poor social functioning, poor housing, inadequate state-supported child-care, illiteracy, unemployment, and excessive alcohol consumption may all contribute to violence in the family. Families where both partners are handicapped need regular social supervision.

Organic brain syndromes

The organic dementias are a rare cause of dangerous behaviour. They include senile and pre-senile organic psychosis, alcoholic psychosis, alcoholic dementia (Korsakov's psychosis), drug psychoses, and transient organic psychotic conditions. These disorders are characterized by confusion, disorientation, memory loss, poor concentration, lack of judgement, and sometimes hallucinations. Most people with severe memory loss require institutional care. For example, a man with an alcoholic dementia could play the piano and converse reasonably convincingly, but could not remember who he was, where he was, or what he had said a few minutes earlier. Unpredictably, when in hospital, he killed the man in the next bed. He had no memory of the incident, and was found unfit to plead at his trial. He had never been violent before; but when assessing his potential for future violence caution needed to be exercised, and it was concluded that, as his condition was untreatable and his mental state unchanged, he represented a risk to other patients. He is detained in Broadmoor Hospital under the Criminal Procedure (Insanity) Act 1964.

The brain-damaged patient is usually a young male with a frontal lobe syndrome following a road-traffic accident. He has intellectual impairment and memory loss, and often demonstrates disinhibited behaviour. He is usually mobile, and may make inappropriate sexual advances to women, which include touching, indecent exposure, and improper suggestions. Violence is uncommon but, when it does occur, is usually minor. Patients with organic brain disorders are often childish, and have a lowered tolerance of frustration.

Epilepsy is not associated with an increased tendency to violent behaviour. The concept of the 'epileptic personality' has been discredited. It used to be thought that persons suffering from epilepsy were more likely to be irritable and aggressive. Violent incidents do, rarely, occur in epileptic fugue states, when patients are in an altered state of consciousness. They may be able to perform motor activities like driving a car, but, afterwards, have no recollection of what they have done during that period.

TREATMENT AND MANAGEMENT OF THE MENTALLY DISORDERED VIOLENT OFFENDER

General approach

Psychiatric treatment incorporates the skills of doctors, nurses, psychologists, occupational therapists, and, perhaps most important, the family and the patient. There is no cure for schizophrenia, and little scientific understanding of its cause or causes. Schizophrenia cannot be prevented; but the effects of the illness can be modified. Depressive illness can be treated successfully with antidepressant drugs, and the duration of the illness can be dramatically reduced. However, in most cases it is not possible to predict whether the illness will recur. Thus, psychiatric treatment can broadly be seen as encompassing everything that happens to a patient between diagnosis and recovery and post-recovery.

The diagnosis is of crucial importance, and the doctor must take a thorough history of the illness, the presenting symptoms, the personal and family background, any previous medical and psychiatric treatment (including drug and alcohol use), and any violence or offending behaviour. While eliciting the history she or he will be observing the appearance, the behaviour, and the demeanour of the patient. Even if the patient says nothing, or is too restless to be interviewed, a provisional diagnosis should be attempted, and arrangements should be made for further assessment and treatment. This is usually referred to as 'management'. The final diagnosis may not be arrived at immediately, but as full an assessment as possible should be made. What is wrong with the patient? How long has something been wrong? Why is he or she behaving like this? Who can provide more information about the patient's background and history? Is the patient under the influence of alcohol or drugs? Has the patient a history of psychiatric illness? Has the patient a record of violence, and in what context? Could this be an organic as opposed to a functional psychosis? This may seem a tall order when confronted in casualty or in the police station by an excited patient; but much of this information will be obtained at a glance. Or the patient may be accompanied by a relative or the police, who will tell you what they know.

However disturbed or threatening a patient may seem, there is usually a part of that person in touch with reality. There is a condition known as catatonic schizophrenia, where the patient is completely withdrawn, mute, and inaccessible; but this is not common. It is important to approach patients the right way, and to explain who one is and that one wants to help. Sometimes small gestures are more important than words: perhaps offering the patient a seat or something to drink. It is often appropriate to empathize with what one thinks the patient may be experiencing. If patients look suspicious and are guarded in their answers this may be a cue to enquire whether they feel someone is trying to harm them or is talking about them in a pejorative or malevolent way. It is usually not a good idea to try and persuade patients that they are wrong in their beliefs; this inevitably leads to confrontation, which can result in further distress, and sometimes violence.

Social workers have difficult decisions to make about the safety of children, and may themselves be at risk from assaults. Social and other professional workers have been threatened, assaulted, and in some cases killed by people for whom they have had a statutory responsibility. Social workers and others who have contact with aggressive clients should not stay alone in the same room as someone who has threatened violence or shown signs of losing control. It is best to terminate the interview, or to request help from a colleague where this is possible. It is also important to recognize that isolated and inadequate people do become dependent on social workers, nurses, doctors, etc., and occasionally react with violence when the relationship is terminated. Patients and clients have damaged the property of professionals, threatened violence, taken hostages, and caused great fear. It is difficult to assess how dangerous it is for doctors, social workers, nurses, the police, and others to visit disturbed people in their homes. The risk can be minimized by taking sensible precautions (see Chapter 2). It is unwise for any professional with a statutory responsibility for taking children into care, for removing people to hospital, or for detaining under the Mental Health Act, to pursue these objectives while unaccompanied. The disturbed patient, or even someone who is simply angry, will be more reassured by someone who is confident, feels safe, and knows what he or she is doing. It is possible to be compassionate and understanding and at the same time to exercise one's professional duties and responsibilities.

Management of physical violence

The management of the acutely disturbed patient may require physical restraint. Methods of control and restraint have been developed which enable nurses who have been trained in the technique and other professionals to restrain a violent or aggressive patient without causing injury to the patient or to the nursing staff. Once restrained, it is usually necessary to sedate the patient and seclude him until he can safely be reintegrated into the ward. Seclusion is used only when absolutely necessary, and never as a punishment. Patients in conditions of seclusion need constant observation, and accurate records must be kept. Dangerous objects which could be used as weapons should be removed, and precautions taken to ensure that the patients cannot harm themselves. When patients are not responsible or in control of their behaviour, a few hours in seclusion, adequate medication, and good nursing care can help them much more than allowing them their freedom, which may result in dangerous behaviour and injuries to other patients and staff.

Disturbed patients in the casualty departments of hospitals and in police stations present special problems. Patients may be brought in by the police or wander in unaccompanied. They may be aggressive or noisy or both. They are probably incapable of giving an account of themselves, and may resent any questioning. They may be injured or smell of alcohol, and professional staff have to make a provisional diagnosis and decide what to do. If the patient is thought to be suffering from a psychiatric disorder, the police surgeon in a police station, or the duty psychiatrist in a general hospital, should be asked for advice. Preparations may need to be made for the patient's detention under the Mental Health Act, and this will involve contacting an Approved Social Worker and (where possible) the patient's general practitioner. The general practitioner or police surgeon will request advice from the duty psychiatrist. Immediate treatment can be given under common law, and it is often sensible once the diagnosis has been made to give an injection of a major tranquillizer to sedate the patient. This should not be done unless an organic cause of the patient's behaviour has been excluded. Barbiturates are contraindicated, and can be dangerous when used to sedate patients, who may, for example, have taken an overdose of alcohol or narcotic drugs.

In the police station there may be concern about restraining and secluding a psychiatric patient. This is understandable, as a police cell is not an appropriate 'place of safety'. Under Section 136 of the Mental Health Act the police may remove a person thought to be suffering from a mental disorder and considered in need of care or control to a place of safety. Unfortunately, the 'place of safety' is all too often a police station. Most psychiatric hospitals have no reception facilities, and disturbed psychiatric patients are either taken to general hospital casualty departments or to police stations. This is not the fault of the police, who would much prefer to take the mentally disordered to psychiatric hospitals. The person may be detained in the place of safety for up to 72 hours. The purpose of Section 136 is to enable the person to be examined by a doctor and interviewed by an Approved Social Worker. The Home Office Circular 66/90 recommends that the place of safety should be a hospital rather than a police station. Attention has been drawn to the numbers of persons admitted to hospital in England and Wales under Section 136, but these do not include cases where the person was taken to a police station as a place of safety and either admitted to hospital under another provision of the Mental Health Act or detained elsewhere. In 1991, attention was drawn to the disproportionate use of the powers of the Mental Health Act in cases of members of minority ethnic communities, especially Afro-Caribbeans.

Psychiatric provision

The psychiatric services comprise the district psychiatric hospital and community services, the regional forensic psychiatry services, including regional secure units, and the special hospitals. The district psychiatric services provide a comprehensive service for the majority of psychiatric patients. A minority of patients need nursing in conditions of physical security. Whether patients need security depends on whether they are likely to abscond from an open ward, whether they have demonstrated any serious violence recently or in the past, and whether they are thought to represent a risk in terms of violent behaviour. Physical security can be perimeter security, ward security, or room security, or a mixture of all these. It is important to remember that patients cannot be treated if they are not there. A locked door may be all that is required to detain the patients physically so that they can benefit from medical and nursing care. The general rule is that patients should be nursed in the least restrictive environment compatible with the patient's safety and the safety of others. In the past the 'locked ward' had a bad reputation, which in many cases was justified. These wards were overcrowded and understaffed, and there was little creative therapy to occupy the patients.

Psychiatric hospitals

In the 1960s and 1970s the conditions in some psychiatric hospitals were the subject of public enquiries. The subsequent reports were highly critical, and described a lamentable lack of care and cruel and inhumane treatments. At the same time hospital beds were closing, and the long stay population of hospitals was moved into the community. Joint finance was established to promote the transfer of resources from the Health Service to local authorities to provide community facilities for the discharged mentally ill. In the 1970s there was a scandal when it was discovered that patients were being transferred from mental hospitals to boarding houses at English seaside resorts. These patients had no psychiatric supervision, and had to fend for themselves in a deprived and sometimes hostile environment. The position in the 1990s is not much improved for the discharged mentally ill, who continue to drift to inner-city areas, where they live in hotels and hostels for single homeless people. A very high psychiatric morbidity has been found in the single homeless living in voluntary-aided accommodation.

The mentally ill are a vulnerable and dependent group. They have no political clout, and historically the only improvements in the care of the mentally ill have come about as a result of scandals. The current scandal is the number of mentally disordered offenders in prisons. Suicides in prison are rising, and most at risk are young males with multiple handicaps and young males with schizophrenia. Five to 10 per cent of the remand and sentenced population are persons who need to be in hospital, and between 20 per cent and 30 per cent are mentally disordered in a broader sense. This latter group may be addicted to drugs or alcohol, and are usually socially deprived and of low intellect.

The closure of psychiatric hospitals and the reduction in numbers of beds has had a profound effect on the quality of the psychiatric services offered to patients. Acute admission wards are reluctant to admit the chronically mentally ill population who are now in the community. As a result these patients remain in the community, and, as their illnesses deteriorate, a proportion will fall foul of the law. Once in the criminal justice system it may be very difficult to reintroduce them into the largely open conditions in psychiatric hospitals. These hospitals are also reluctant to admit any patients who show assaultive or violent tendencies.

Regional secure units

In 1974 the Home Office and DHSS published a report of the committee on mentally abnormal offenders, which proposed the immediate development of secure units within each regional health authority. In the same year the report of the working party on security in NHS psychiatric hospitals stated that there were 2000 patients in NHS psychiatric facilities who required security.

It was hoped that regional secure units would take patients from special hospitals and from the courts and prisons, and so reduce the numbers of patients inappropriately placed. Although the report of the working party on security in NHS psychiatric hospitals had identified 2000 patients, the target number of regional secure unit beds was 1000. This target has not been reached, and in 1991 there were only about 600 regional secure unit beds. The demand for secure beds is about double what has been provided. In order to reduce the numbers of mentally disordered people in prisons and special hospitals, each region will need to have of the order of 40 beds per million population.

Regional secure units are of varying size. The largest unit is in the West Midlands, with 100 beds. The optimum size for a secure unit is probably 40 to 80 beds. Secure units are relatively well staffed, and an average 15-bedded secure unit will have one consultant, one senior registrar, two occupational therapists, one social worker, and 30 nursing staff. This level of staffing enables patients to receive individual treatment in a calm and therapeutic environment.

Special hospitals

Special hospitals are constituted by Section 4 of the National Health Service Act 1977, by which the Secretary of State for Social Services is required to provide special hospitals 'for patients subject to detention' who 'require treatment under conditions of special security on account of their dangerous, violent and criminal propensities'. In 1989 the management of the special hospitals was reorganized, and a new Special Hospitals Health Authority was constituted. The Special Hospitals Health Authority manages the three special hospitals,

Broadmoor, Rampton, and Ashworth; but each hospital has its own local management. The reorganization of the management of special hospitals has introduced general management, and each special hospital has a general manager responsible to the Special Hospitals Health Authority.

Broadmoor Hospital was opened in 1863, following the second Criminal Lunatics Act in 1860, which was introduced to make better provision for the custody and care of mentally disordered offenders. Patients who were found not guilty on the grounds of insanity or were found insane, were ordered to be detained in custody 'at Her Majesty's pleasure'. Patients were also admitted from prisons when found to be mentally disordered on remand and while serving sentences. The criteria for admission to a special hospital are that the patient should suffer from a mental disorder as defined in the Mental Health Act 1983 and should be considered to represent a grave and immediate danger to the public.

Patients in special hospitals suffer from one of the four forms of mental disorder as defined in the Mental Health Act 1983. In Broadmoor Hospital 75 per cent of the patients are classified as suffering from mental illness and 25 per cent are classified as suffering from psychopathic disorder. In Rampton Hospital 50 per cent of the patients suffer from mental illness, 21 per cent from psychopathic disorder, and the remainder from mental impairment and severe mental impairment. There is a preponderance of males in special hospitals, in a ratio of 4:1. All the patients in special hospitals are detained patients. At Broadmoor Hospital 60 per cent of the patients are subject to special restrictions, and can only be discharged by a Tribunal or by the Secretary of State.

The treatments available in special hospitals are as good as if not better than, those found in regional secure units and psychiatric hospitals. The perimeter security allows patients more freedom to move from their wards to the workshops and the occupations department. Although security is higher in special hospitals the atmosphere for the patients is less oppressive than the ward security of regional secure units.

LEGAL ASPECTS OF MANAGEMENT

It has been estimated that about a third of sentenced prisoners suffer from some form of mental disorder. This includes persons suffering from alcoholism and drug abuse. These figures might lead one to suppose that the legal system does not make provision for transfer or diversion of these offenders from the criminal justice system.

The truth is rather different. The mentally disordered are in prison because there are inadequate resources for them in hospitals or in the community.

Example: A 67-year-old man caused £500 000 worth of damage by setting fire to a building. He was unkempt and apparently used to sleeping rough. The police could not get much useful information from him. He was remanded in custody, and a week later he was seen by a psychiatrist, who diagnosed schizophrenia. The psychiatrist recommended that the court order a psychiatric report so that the man could be seen by a psychiatrist from the district psychiatric hospital. Three weeks after the original remand, the court were unable to order a psychiatric report as he was not able to plead. He was remanded for a further week in custody, and, when he appeared in court the next week, it was suggested that the prison medical officer should request a psychiatric opinion. Three weeks later a report was prepared by the prison medical officer reporting that the accused was unfit to plead. There was no psychiatric report from the catchment area psychiatrist. The case continues, and this 67-year-old mentally ill man remains in prison. What should have been done? Although the offence was serious in terms of the amount of damage caused, there is no suggestion that this patient needed special security. He should have been admitted to the local psychiatric hospital when first arrested. The police would have agreed to his being detained under a treatment section of the Mental Health Act in the catchment area psychiatric hospital. They would then have been able to decide whether to proceed with a prosecution. Difficulties arise in cases like this because of the reluctance of psychiatric hospitals to admit patients who are of no fixed abode and who may, become a long-term commitment. As the National Health Service reforms take effect, it may be even more difficult to admit patients of no fixed abode who may, or may not, have had a history of treatment in other districts or regions. An alternative for this patient would have been admission to a psychiatric hospital as a condition of his bail. Unfortunately the remand sections (Sections 35 and 36) are not very helpful in this particular case. As the charge is one which is only punishable in the Crown Court, the Magistrates Court cannot make an order under Section 35: a Section 36 order can only be made in the Crown Court. A section 35 order has another disadvantage, in that patients are not subject to the consent to treatment provision of the Mental Health Act 1983, and cannot be given treatment without consent. It might conceivably be possible to arrange a hearing in the Crown Court; but this would be exceptional. The best way of dealing with this man would clearly have been to admit him to hospital under a civil section, and to leave the police to decide about prosecution.

The Mental Health Act 1983

While most patients are admitted informally, the Mental Health Act makes provision for the compulsory detention of patients suffering from any of the four forms of mental disorder as defined in the Act. Admission to hospital can be for assessment or for treatment, and there is provision for the detention of patients who are already in hospital. Admissions for assessment are for 72 hours and, where two doctors make a recommendation under Section 2, for 28 days. Admission for treatment (Section 3) allows a patient to be admitted to a hospital and detained for a period of six months. The grounds for admission under the Mental Health Act are that the patient is suffering from one of the four forms of mental disorder of a nature or degree which makes it appropriate for him to receive treatment in hospital; and it is necessary for the health or safety of the patient or for the protection of other persons that he should receive such treatment. In the case of psychopathic disorder or mental impairment the doctors have to confirm that treatment is likely to alleviate or prevent a deterioration of the patient's condition.

The Mental Health Act 1983 included recommendations made by the Butler Committee (1974) with the introduction of the remand sections. Section 35 empowers the court to remand an accused to hospital for a report. Section 36 allows the Crown Court to remand an accused to hospital for treatment.

Hospital orders (Section 37, Mental Health Act 1983) can be made in the Magistrates Court and the Crown Court. The Magistrates Court can in certain circumstances make a hospital order without recording a conviction. In most cases a hospital order is made in the Magistrates Court following conviction on lesser charges and in the Crown Court following conviction on more serious charges. The hospital order is the most frequently used section for the detention of mentally disordered offenders. If the safety of the public is thought to be at risk the court can apply a restriction order under Section 41. The restriction order makes the patient liable to be detained in hospital unless absolutely discharged by a Mental Health Review Tribunal or by the Secretary of State. Restriction orders can be for a limited period or without limit of time.

There are also provisions under the Mental Health Act for the transfer by the Home Office of remand and sentenced prisoners to hospital for treatment. There has been some concern expressed about the transfer of sentenced prisoners to hospital towards the end of their sentence. Once transferred to hospital, the person concerned then finds himself subject to what can be indeterminate detention.

Patients' rights

A patient detained under the Mental Health Act has a right to apply to a Mental Health Review Tribunal for his discharge except where the order for detention is for 72 hours. Mental Health Review Tribunals were established in 1960 following the introduction of the Mental Health Act 1959. The Tribunal is appointed by the Lord Chancellor, and consists of a legal, a medical, and a lay member. Medical members are usually psychiatrists, and the Tribunal is chaired by the legal member. In the case of a restricted patient the legal member is drawn from a panel of specially appointed lawyers, who are usually circuit judges or recorders. Patients are entitled to legal advice, and solicitors may obtain the services of an independent psychiatrist to prepare a report. The Tribunal also obtains a medical report from the patient's responsible medical officer, who usually represents the detaining authority at the hearing. The medical member of the Tribunal examines the patient before the hearing, and both he and the independent psychiatrist have access to the patient's medical records. At the hearing the Tribunal has powers to discharge unrestricted patients, and to discharge restricted patients conditionally or absolutely. Patients who have been transferred from prison and who are subject to a restriction order cannot be discharged by a Tribunal. The Tribunal can make recommendations to the Secretary of State concerning its view as to whether the patient should be returned to prison or should remain in hospital for further treatment.

Patients have no right to refuse medication during the first three months following detention, but after that it is unlawful to give patients medication without their informed consent. If it is felt to be in the interests of the patient to continue with medication, a second opinion can be obtained from a doctor appointed by the Mental Health Act Commission. Electro-convulsive therapy cannot be given to a patient without either his consent or a second opinion.

Mental Health Act Commission

Between 1959 and 1983 there was no statutory independent body designated to visit psychiatric hospitals and to protect the interests of patients. During this period there were a succession of scandals and allegations of ill-treatment, cruelty, and neglect. The Mental Health Act Commission was established in 1983 as a Special Health Authority, and is responsible to the Secretary of State for Health. It is an independent body with a chairman and 91 part-time members.

The functions of the Commission are laid down in section 121 of the Mental Health Act 1983.

The role of the Home Office and the protection of the public

The Home Office is responsible for ordering the transfers of remand and sentenced prisoners to hospital and for the supervision of conditionally discharged restricted patients. This latter function is administered through C3 Division of the Home Office, and officials remain in close contact with both the patient's responsible medical officer and the social worker who is managing the patient in the community. Regular reports are submitted to the Home Office, who have the right to recall a patient to hospital at any time. The Home Office usually only exercises its right to recall if there is a serious risk to the safety of the public. Once recalled to hospital, a patient has the right to apply to a Mental Health Review Tribunal.

The Home Office may also commission the advice of the Advisory Board on restricted patients. This is an independent non-statutory body whose members are appointed by the Home Secretary. The Advisory Board was set up in 1973 following a report chaired by Sir Carl Aarvold which reviewed the procedures for the discharge and supervision of psychiatric patients subject to restriction. The Aarvold Committee considered that there were patients in special hospitals who, because of the nature of their offending, did require special care in assessing their suitability for conditional discharge. The selection of cases is made by officials in the Home Office, who seek the agreement of the Minister concerned that the case should be referred to the Advisory Board.

Diversion of mentally disordered offenders from custody

In 1990 the Home Office issued Circular 66/90 entitled 'Provision for Mentally Disordered Offenders' to encourage a policy of diversion of mentally disordered offenders from custody. Circular 66/90 was circulated to health authorities, social services, the probation service, and Magistrates and Crown Courts. Circular 66/90 recognized that diversion from custody could occur at a number of different stages in the criminal justice process, and made recommendations about a multidisciplinary approach to the problem. Court liaison services have been set up in various parts of the country to study the size of the problem and to initiate procedures aimed at diverting the mentally disordered from the criminal justice system to hospital.

PREDICTING AND PREVENTING VIOLENCE

The best predictor of future dangerousness is a previous history of dangerous behaviour. Dangerousness can be defined as violence involving injury or lasting psychological harm. It is easier to predict that someone will repeat a violent act if he has shown a tendency to behave in a similar way on previous occasions. If a man habitually becomes aggressive when drunk, it is reasonably safe to assume that while he continues to drink to excess he will present a danger. On the other hand, if someone has committed a single offence involving violence and has otherwise been a stable person, the statistical chances of a repetition must be small unless there are other factors, including mental disorder, which might influence the prediction. Predicting violence in patients suffering from psychotic disorders is much easier than predicting whether a sex offender will commit a further sexual offence or whether an arsonist will reoffend. Some patients who suffer from schizophrenia are unpredictably violent and show no premonitory signs. These patients are more dangerous than patients who make clear statements about their victims and what they intend doing.

Example: A 26-year-old man with a history of admission to psychiatric hospitals had a diagnosis of schizophrenia. Following his last admission he remained rather solitary, and was unemployed. He lived with his mother and sister, and had never shown any violence. On the day of the offence he was watching his sister peel potatoes and suddenly became convinced that she was stealing his brain. He got up, walked into the kitchen, picked up a knife, and stabbed his sister to death. Following this he could give no other explanation for killing other than that he felt an uncontrollable urge to stab her. This patient did recover to some extent; but because of the unpredictable nature of his violence he will be difficult to supervise.

Example: A 25-year-old woman was diagnosed as suffering from schizophrenia at the age of 16. During the previous nine years she had spent several months each year in hospital. Following discharge from hospital she had not taken her medication and her illness had relapsed. Each admission to hospital was precipitated by some form of violence involving her stabbing or attempting to stab her family or strangers. As she had not caused any serious harm she was not considered to be particularly dangerous. This was an error of judgement: a patient suffering from schizophrenia who attacks or threatens people with knives is a considerable danger to the public. She was admitted to Broadmoor Hospital after stabbing a stranger in the street. Following treatment in Broadmoor Hospital she has made an excellent recovery; but, while it may be appropriate to recommend her transfer from conditions of maximum security, caution must be exercised before recommending her discharge to the community.

All those concerned with the care of the mentally disordered in hospital and in the community are conscious of their need to protect the public. The supervision of psychiatric patients is of the utmost importance, and social workers, psychiatrists, families, and in some case the Home Office work together to minimize the risk to the public by providing adequate support, close supervision, and regular assessments of the patient's mental state.

Psychiatrists and others who are asked to make predictions about dangerousness have no reliable scientific tools to help them. At best, predictions are made on the basis of statistical evidence – for example, the reconviction rate of sex offenders; but statistics will not give an accurate prediction in any individual case.

Example: A 30-year-old man had convictions for indecent exposure during his early teens, and at the age of 17 indecently exposed himself to a woman, who retaliated by attacking him with a rake. He claimed he lost his temper, pushed her to the ground, put his hands around her throat until she lost consciousness, and after undoing her trousers ran off. He was convicted of attempted rape, and after serving a three-year prison sentence committed no further offences for five years. He then committed a series of offences involving breaking into houses where young women were asleep on their own, indecently exposing himself to them while wearing a mask, and then waking them up by indecently assaulting them and masturbating over them. He could give no explanation for this behaviour, and did his best to distance himself from any sexual motive. This man had been committing similar offences since the age of 16, which is evidence that he does have serious sexual psychopathology. There is certainly a risk that he will reoffend when released from prison, but it is impossible to make an accurate prediction. It is also difficult to know whether treatment for his sexual deviation can be expected to minimize the risk.

People who care for disturbed and sometimes violent members of society need support and respect. They put themselves at risk and are responsible for the safety of others. This responsibility is easier to shoulder if the professional can feel confident that his work is being scrutinized by his peers and by other disciplines. He must always be aware of the dangers of professional isolation. Multidisciplinary teams can work well, particularly where members of the team making decisions are of equal of seniority.

FURTHER READING

Dooley, E. (1990). Prison suicide in England and Wales 1972–1987. *British Journal of Psychiatry*, **156**, 40–5.

Glancy, J. (1974). *Revised report of the Working Party on Security in NHS psychiatric hospitals.* DHSS, London.

Gostin, L. (1985). *Secure provision.* Tavistock Publications, London.

Gunn J. Robertson, G., and Dell, S. (1988). *Psychiatric aspects of imprisonment. Criminal statistics for England and Wales.* Academic Press, London.

Home Office and DHSS (1975). *Report of the Committee on Mentally Abnormal Offenders (Butler Report).* HMSO, London. Mental Health Act (1983). HMSO, London.

Taylor, P.J. and Gunn, J. (1984). Violence and psychosis I – Risk of violence among psychotic men. *British Medical Journal* **288**, 1945–9.

Working for patients. *Provision for mentally disordered offenders*, Home Office Circular 66/90. Home office, London.

5 The care of victims

Gillian Mezey and Jonathan Shepherd

The effects of assault range from a temporary crisis of loss of confidence in one's professional abilities, humiliation, and days off work to prolonged psychological disturbance – including depression, generalized and phobic anxiety, and the maladaptive use of coping strategies, including drugs and alcohol, to contain feelings of anxiety and distress. In an extreme form, individual victims, may then themselves be unable to function in a therapeutic way, and thus will be forced to cease employment.

Violence at work has repercussions, and not only for the victim. It may affect the assailant in terms of prolonged detention under the Mental Health Act, or arrest and prosecution and custody. It affects colleagues and the health-care team, leading to a decrease in morale and economic loss through absenteeism. Clearly, prevention of violence to staff in the first place is required to obviate the need for the treatment of victims. Although health workers are most at risk from the public, the risk of aggression from fellow workers should not be forgotten. Insidious forms of violence at work include sexual harassment and sexual and racial discrimination. This 'violence' is subtle and pernicious, and more difficult to identify, monitor, and control, probably because of its often subtle nature and the fact that in many cases it is merely a manifestation of the prevailing subculture that both promotes it and colludes in it at the expense of selected individuals.

Treating victims of assault must start by preventing violence: risk factors need to be identified, which means monitoring assaults and collecting data about who hits, who is hit, when it occurs, what the precipitating features are, and what the victim's as well as the victimizer's perceptions are of the incident (see Chapter 2). Where the patient is known, a history of aggression is the best prediction of future aggression, and patients with a history of aggression can be identified as potential assailants. Frequent changes in staffing may predispose to violence, particularly in primary-care settings and psychiatric wards, because they lead to inconsistent and unstable care. A recent study found that nurses least familiar with patients were assaulted most often. A study of violence in the Accident and Emergency Department found that nurses were most at risk of assault and receptionists least so, and that assailants grabbed any nearby object as a weapon. The development of uncluttered treatment areas, with fitted furniture where practicable, and careful staffing allocation at times when assaults are most likely are important steps in preventing violence.

Information about potential aggression needs to be communicated effectively to all staff in order to prevent assault. All staff must know of risk situations in order to avoid them. Inexperienced staff are more liable to be hit, perhaps because, in a hierarchical work structure, it is the inexperienced junior staff who are least likely to read safety-at-work codes of practice and regulations, and therefore to find themselves in situations they should have avoided.

Certain individuals may be more vulnerable to assault. A question often asked is whether patients are more likely to be assaultive to men or women. Certain patients may be calmed by a female health worker; others may find one provocative. Preventive measures should be considered in terms of individual, situational, structural, or managerial factors. The presence of adequate alarm systems placed where the patients are known to have a potential for violence, for instance in urban priority areas and in Casualty Departments, is essential. Alarm systems must be accessible and easy to respond to, otherwise they are useless. If patients are known to be unpredictable or dangerous, simple measures such as questioning them about their possession of weapons may be useful in pre-empting violence. Where patients are suspected of carrying weapons, it is reasonable to ask them if they would agree to being searched. Concerns about dangerousness should always be communicated to others, and feelings of uncertainty about particular patients should be taken seriously rather than dismissed as a merely subjective concern. Simple straightforward structural changes that can avoid assault include placing the desk and chair near to an exit, ensuring that the exit cannot be blocked by the patient, avoiding or being aware of blind corners and structures that obstruct clear views in a health-centre or ward, and the provision of adequate lighting. Environments that are bland, dull, and shabby indicate a lack of respect for the patients, who may in turn demonstrate a lack of respect for their environment and carers in the form of aggression and violent behaviour (see Chapter 2). Significantly, substantial progress has been made to prevent, bar violence by regular redecoration and furnishing and paying attention to producing a peaceful 'atmosphere'.

CONTROL AND RESTRAINT

Control and restraint works on the assumption that aggressive patients should be dealt with 'physically' only as a last resort. The aim of control and restraint techniques is to increase skills in defusing or de-escalating potentially violent behaviour and in preventing physical injury to both parties. The most effective and safe way to deal with a physically assaultive patient for both carer and patients is to 'escape', until an effective and controlled response can be organized. There is some evidence that staff properly trained in aggression-control techniques experience fewer assaults than their untrained colleagues and are less likely to sustain a physical injury as a result (see Chapter 2).

CARE OF THE VICTIM

Staff who are assaulted should not instantly acquire the status of a patient, although they often do. Reactions of fellow-workers range from being over-protective to being indifferent, critical, hostile, and blaming.

An adequate complaints procedure is essential. Monitoring assaults in a Health Centre can convey an important message and is in itself therapeutic: that assault is a problem for *everyone*, that the victim's experience is taken seriously, that the assault is likely to lead to certain psychological problems, and that efforts are being made to contain violence. Merely 'talking through' the incident to someone who appears to be listening and taking the experience seriously can help alleviate distress and anxiety, and may prevent prolonged distress and maladaptive coping reactions from developing. The majority of health workers who are assaulted recover from the experience and are able to resume work, albeit with some adaptation in their behaviour and often some alteration in their feelings about themselves and in their attitude to work.

At the simplest level, treatment can be provided by both formal and informal support structures, the latter meaning the expression of sympathy from colleagues and sensitive handling which may be all that the victim wants or requires. A study of assaulted nurses emphasized the importance of taking time to talk about the assault, of hearing people to check up whether victims are all right, of some 'time off', and of some breathing space to be allowed for victims to regain composure and to 'process' what has just occurred. A number commented on the need to be taught coping mechanisms, to deal both with the assault and with the feelings that arose subsequently.

However, in spite of the difficulties experienced by many victims of assault at work, very few receive any counselling afterwards. In spite of medicine being a caring profession, there exists an ethic of stoicism, a view that health professionals should not complain and are expected to put up with any hardship, as if nurses and doctors should accept violence, assault, and abuse as part of their job descriptions.

The needs of health-service employees are no different from those of victims of violence in general. Following assault they may require medical attention, crisis counselling, legal advice, and information regarding compensation and their rights.

After initial management of physical injuries, the victim requires reassurance about his/her current physical safety, reassurance that the assault has been taken seriously, reassurance that he/she is not being blamed, and reassurance about his/her professional skill and capabilities. Victims of assault need the opportunity to talk about what happened. This can be at the level of peer support; but it is also essential that assaulted health workers, who are often in junior positions, should receive support and encouragement from senior colleagues and management. Failure to provide this leads to a sense of injustice, betrayal, and alienation from the workplace.

If necessary, the victim may need time away from the work environment for hours or days, depending on the seriousness of the assault. A system of peer support has been developed in the United States, where health workers form a 'buddy' system with another team and so provide support for assaulted colleagues. Although the effects of such a scheme are difficult to evaluate, initial audit appeared to show a slowing down in staff turnover and a decrease in absenteeism.

In general, it is important to have built-in support structures for health workers, particularly in circumstances where levels of violence are high and assault is frequent – to create an ethos that states that it is 'all right' and expected that staff will be stressed much of the time and that violence is an additional source of stress that may precipitate a crisis in the victim.

MANAGEMENT OF PHYSICAL INJURIES

Management of physical injuries should follow the same course in health-care workers as in any other group of patients, though confidentiality and privacy are particularly important, and management outside the victim's place of work may be necessary. It is also necessary to make sure that health-care professionals understand their injuries, the treatment that is required, and long-term effects; it is easy to assume, mistakenly, that all health-care professionals understand the detailed implications of all injuries. For example, glib explanations that all that is necessary is a speedy Gillies lift will be meaningless to all but maxillofacial surgeons familiar with surgical techniques for the treatment of fractured cheek bones. Similarly, dental practitioners may not be familiar with the effects of potentially devastating hand injuries or the terminology associated with their management.

Health-care professionals develop means of communicating with patients which depend on particular patterns of speech and facial expressions. These may not be possible after even a fairly minor facial injury. A numb lip or a black eye will interfere with effective communication with patients. It is important that health-care workers are reassured that such afflictions normally resolve within a few weeks. Acknowledgement of the effects of such injuries, even leaving aside hand injuries which affect function, may necessitate several days or weeks away from patient contact. Rehabilitation after facial injury is particularly important for health-care professionals, as it is for other workers whose livelihood and effectiveness depends upon highly developed communication skills.

Management of facial injuries

The management of minor abrasions and bruises should follow normal lines, and attention to detail is essential in the repair of lacerations either with sutures or adhesive dressings. Management of fractures of the facial bones is often conservative; but a soft diet and adequate pain-relief will always be necessary following a fractured jaw. A broken nose will require thorough assessment, particularly to assess bruising around the nasal septum. An operation may be necessary, which may be performed under local anaesthesia on an out-patient basis. Various methods of holding the broken nose in place are available, and include obvious and disfiguring 'T'-shaped nasal plasters and packing of the nose with ribbon gauze.

Broken cheek-bones may require repositioning if they are displaced. The usual way of doing this is to slide an instrument underneath the cheek-bone from a small incision made above the hairline. The cheek-bone is then levered into its correct position, following which it may require no further stabilization. In some instances, the cheek bone may need to be held rigidly in place with a metal plate, which is most often inserted through a small incision at the outer aspect of the eyebrow. Later assessment of the recovery from double vision may be necessary and attendance at Eye Clinics as well at Oral Surgery and ENT Clinics may be necessary. The management of severe facial injuries is often multidisciplinary in nature and it is important to co-ordinate visits to hospital so that time-consuming and expensive multiple visits are avoided.

The treatment of jaw fractures has been revolutionized over the past ten years by the use of small metal plates to hold the pieces together. This treatment has largely replaced the traditional wiring of the jaws, in which the jaws are wired solidly together for a period of up to six weeks. The metal plates which are used for fixation of jaw fractures are inserted through small incisions, usually inside the mouth. As also happens with broken cheek-bones, these metal plates are often left in place, though occasionally they become infected and need to be removed under a second general anaesthetic; but this later removal is often carried out on a day-case basis.

Dental treatment

Teeth are often damaged or knocked out in an assault. Particularly for health-care professionals in contact with patients on a regular basis, dental treatment of a high standard is necessary. Such treatment is nearly always best carried out by a dental practitioner away from a hospital; though dental specialists who are experts in fillings, crowns, and dentures are increasingly employed in hospitals.

Management of other injuries

The management of any injury includes prompt assessment and appropriate treatment. This book is not the place for detailed descriptions of the physical effects and management of stab wounds of the chest or abdomen or of injuries brought about by firearms. Facial injuries are by far the most frequent in assault, and hand injuries are the next most frequent, though comparatively rare. The management of hand injuries should include assessment of function and nerve damage, so that repair of tendons and nerves can be carried out at the optimum time. Thorough assessment at an early stage is required, not least so that detailed descriptions of all injuries and treatment can be included in compensation claims.

Health-care professionals may find the process of the assessment and management of physical injuries trying and frustrating; but this needs to be carried out in an unhurried way, with all necessary special investigations such as X-rays. All health-care professionals should be sensitive to the needs of colleagues. It is dangerous to assume that they are somehow immune from injury or from its effects, and particularly that they are somehow to blame for getting injured.

CRISIS INTERVENTION

Crisis intervention is a particularly useful exercise for victims of assault. This form of counselling operates on the assumption that the victim was 'normal' before the assault, that assault precipitates a state of crisis or disequilibrium, and that a return to a normal state occurs after counselling. Crisis counselling comprises no more than twelve sessions; but often only one or two sessions are all that is required to put the assault into perspective and to restore a crucial sense of control to the victim. A one-off 'chat' *may* be enough. But the victim of assault often continues to remember the incident and fears its repetition long after colleagues have forgotten, or believe that he or she should have 'got over it'.

A crucial part of crisis counselling is the opportunity to describe, not only what has happened, but one's feelings in detail, without being criticized, ridiculed, or negatively judged. The victim will also require negative or distorted views arising from the assault to be corrected, such as 'I was assaulted because I am a bad nurse', 'I was assaulted because I didn't take care', or 'I was assaulted because I am a vulnerable person.' The assault needs to be discussed and put into perspective, and responsibility for what has happened needs to be appropriately attributed to the assaulter. Successful processing of the experience should lead to the victim's regaining a sense of control over her or his professional and personal life.

Opportunities for counselling should be provided within the working environment, although it should be remembered that because of the 'hierarchy' that exists professionally, it may be difficult, particularly for junior health-workers, to be open and direct about their feelings. They may wish to express ambivalence, particularly towards their line manager, who may ultimately be responsible for their continuing employment and promotion prospects. Victims fear that they will be regarded as weak and emotionally unstable by their colleagues, so that their career will be jeopardized. By the same token it is often difficult for senior staff, including doctors, to receive support following an assault, because of their difficulties in admitting or acknowledging their own vulnerability and occasional helplessness.

It is therefore important for all health-care facilities to develop links with outside organizations and groups who have special training in recognizing and dealing with the after-effects of violence and crime, such as the national charity Victim Support (see Appendix for contact details).

SPECIFIC TREATMENT

A number of assault victims fail to survive the assault psychologically, and develop multiple, severe, and persistent stress reactions, including phobic anxiety, generalized anxiety, depression, and post-traumatic stress disorder (see Chapter 1).

The assault may trigger off unresolved distress from previous trauma, which may, over time, have been repressed, until its reactivation by later victimization.

A victim's reaction may seem exaggerated and out of proportion to the severity of the assault, and colleagues may feel confused and irritated by the apparent devastations precipitated by an apparently trivial occurrence.

It is important to identify vulnerable individuals at an early stage in order to anticipate prolonged psychological disturbance and to offer appropriate intervention.

Crisis counselling is not enough for victims of assault who experience this form of 'compounded' trauma. Further assessment may be required by the individual's own general practitioner, and referral for specialist psychological and psychiatric help may be necessary. Therapy, when offered, then initially focuses on the current precipitating assault; but the counsellor is likely to move rapidly on to earlier histories of trauma, which may include severe deprivation and sexual and physical abuse. No formal psychiatric treatment should be offered to a victim less than six months after assault, in order to allow natural recovery to take place. After six months, if there is incomplete recovery and continuing problems, the victim is unlikely to make spontaneous readjustment without additional help. Victims of compounded reactions are liable to require more prolonged and specialist care, which should be provided outside the immediate work environment. As has previously been noted, health workers, particularly individuals whose job is to help psychologically disturbed individuals, often find it difficult to recognize their own need for psychological treatment, and may be resistant to suggestions that they are ill or need help. Clearly, unless somebody is willing to accept treatment there is no way that this can or should be forced on them. The following models of therapy have been used extensively and evaluated in the treatment of post-traumatic stress disorder, with victims of assault as well as others.

Chemotherapy

Minor tranquillizers are useful in the immediate management of acute distress, but should be an adjunct to 'talking', and tailed off rapidly to prevent physiological dependence. Anti-depressants may also be useful if clinically indicated.

Behavioural techniques

Behavioural techniques are particularly useful in the treatment of circumscribed symptoms, where the pre-existing personality is relatively unchanged – for example, phobic anxiety and avoidance – and for the correction of disturbed beliefs arising out of the assault.

Systematic desensitization teaches relaxation skills and aims to desensitize fear responses by exposing the victim to a graded series of fear stimuli which he or she must learn to cope with until the stimuli are no longer frightening.

Stress inoculation training (SIT) is based on the premise that by teaching the victim about the nature and origin of fear and anxiety, responses will be modified and controlled. Stress inoculation training consists of a preliminary education phase on the different sorts of reactions to stress. The victim is taught skills to cope with physical and behavioural reactions that arise through high levels of anxiety, for example muscle-relaxation, breath-control, and role-playing. As with most behaviour therapies, the victim is given homework between sessions which rehearses coping skills previously learnt and monitors progress. Behavioural techniques are also helpful in the late alleviation of symptoms of depression, particularly where that depression is associated with guilt, self-criticism, and lowered self-esteem in relation to the assault.

Psychotherapy may be offered in the form of individual or group treatment, and necessarily takes place over a much longer period than either systematic desensitization or stress inoculation training. Psychotherapy is perhaps particularly indicated where the current symptoms are thought to arise from previously unresolved trauma, and where the victim feels that it is not appropriate to use violence at work as a central focus of any treatment programme.

MANAGEMENT RESPONSIBILITY

Clearly management has not only a duty but a vested interest in ensuring the physical safety of employees and in offering appropriate treatment when the system fails them. Failure to provide treatment results in loss of manpower, increases in overtime payments, lowered morale, and increases in fear, and in control issues taking precedence over treatment. Staff who feel unsafe with the people with whom they have daily contact understandably limit their interactions with certain patients. They no longer look forward to coming to work, and demoralization quickly spreads, particularly in a small, tightly-knit health-care team in a health-centre.

So what can and should management do? First, it must ensure that levels of violence at work are consistently and accurately reported. Following any assault, management must ensure immediate physical treatment for the victim, including, if necessary, hospital admission and continuing care. It must consider the question of time off or reallocation, and if necessary should ensure that the victims' friends and families are contacted or that they are accompanied home. Details of particular incidents must be recorded, and patient – assaulters must be interviewed in order to obtain their accounts of assaults. Policies regarding the patient's treatment must be evaluated. Information regarding the assault must be communicated to all staff; and, wherever possible, they should be given the opportunity to discuss and express their feelings about the assault. (see Chapter 2).

The victim will need his or her rights explained, including the mechanism of pursuing any legal action (see Chapter 6). Management generally decide what their view is regarding prosecution, and whether they will support any action taken by the victim. Finally the practice or institution, including the victim of the assault, will need a *post mortem* on the violence, deciding why it happened, whether it could have been prevented, and what further steps should be taken to ensure the safety of all health workers.

There are many sources of help for health-care workers who are assaulted, though continuing care needs to be the province of management because the health-care worker may not be able to summon help or even know what services are available. Trade unions are particularly effective sources of help and representation, and groups such as ambulance staff will find a wealth of services through the Transport Unions. Similarly, NALGO, COHSE, and NUPE (now amalgamated to form 'UNISON') will provide help and advice for many staff. Doctors, dentists, and an increasingly broad spectrum of health-care professionals will find that membership of a defence organization confers benefits in terms of personal injury insurance.

FURTHER READING

Aiken, G.J.M. (1984). Assaults on staff on a locked ward: prediction and consequences. *Medicine, Science, and the Law*, **24**, 199–207.

Engel, F. and Marsh, S. (1986). Helping the employee victim of violence in hospital. *Hospital and Community Psychiatry*, **37** (2), 159–62.

Health Services Advisory Committee. (1987). *Violence to staff in the Health Services*. HMSO, London.

Infantino, J.A. and Musing, S. (1985). Assaults and injuries among staff with and without training in aggression control techniques. *Hospital and Community Psychiatry*, **36** (12), 1312–14.

Lanza, M.L. (1985). How nurses react to patient assaults. *Journal of Psychological Nursing*, **23** (6), 6–10.

Pearson, M., Wilmot, E., and Padi, M. (1986). A study of violent behaviour among inpatients in a psychiatric hospital. *British Journal of Psychiatry*, **149**, 232–5.

Shepherd, J.P. (1990). Victims of personal violence: the relevance of Symond's model of psychological response. *British Journal of Social Work*, **20**, 309–32.

Shepherd, J.P., Shapland, M., Pearce, N.X., *et al.* (1990). Patterns, aetiology and severity of injury in victims of assault. *Journal of the Royal Society of Medicine*, **83**, 75–8.

Shepherd, J.P., Levers, B.G.H., Preston, M., *et al.* (1990). Psychological distress after assaults and accidents. *British Medical Journal*, **301**, 849–50.

Smith, L.J.F. (1987). *Crime in hospitals: diagnosis and prevention*. Crime Prevention Unit, Home Office, London.

Whittington, R. and Wykes, T. (1989). Invisible injury. *Nursing Times*, **42**, 30–2.

6 Compensation for personal injuries caused by crime in the UK

David Miers

INTRODUCTION

The most likely kind of victimization that a health-care worker will suffer is the theft of personal possessions. Despite the headlines, crimes of violence against the person are not that common. In 1990, of 3.7 million offences known to the police, just 6 per cent (240 000) consisted of offences of violence against the person (including sexual offences). Where they do occur, the majority result in no serious injury: of those 240 000 offences, around two-thirds will have caused minor injuries. Nevertheless, some have a greater impact, and for many victims of even minor assaults the impact upon their sense of well-being and of confidence in the world can, at the very least, be temporarily disabling. It is with the possibilities for compensation for the consequences of offences involving personal injury that this chapter is concerned. Theft is not usually accompanied by the use or threat of violence, but where it is, it may be treated by the police as a crime of violence (that is, robbery), and this offence too will be covered in this chapter. Like theft, burglary is a crime against property; but the shock that victims suffer upon discovering that they have been burgled may be no different in its impact upon their well-being than that suffered in consequence of a direct personal assault.

A health-care worker may become the victim of a crime of violence either on or off duty. Where the injury occurs while the worker is on duty, the offender may well be a patient; where it occurs off duty, it is most likely to be just any other offending person. So far as the possibilities for compensation are concerned, these distinctions have little practical importance. Employers have a duty to provide their employees with a safe system of work, and thus where a health-care worker on duty is injured by a patient, it is in theory possible to succeed in a civil action in negligence against a hospital management or a health authority. It would have to be proved that the patient was known to the management or authority to have violent propensities, and that, in the circumstances, they had failed to take reasonable care to contain them and that the worker's injury was closely related to that neglect. There might be liability, for example, where a female nurse is instructed to treat a male patient whose violent propensities are known to the management of the hospital in which he is being compulsory detained under the Mental Health Act 1983, the ward sister having failed first to check that any prescribed drug regime had been complied with. It would certainly be otherwise if a nurse working elsewhere in the hospital were injured following the patient's escape from the constraints normally imposed upon such a person. However, in the analogous context of the prison service, the courts have been reluctant to impose liability upon the management, and such civil action holds out little hope to injured nurses; it would certainly not extend to drunk and violent patients brought into an accident and emergency department.

The same can be said of instances in which health-care workers are attacked by strangers in hostels or other residences managed by the hospital trust or health authority and in which the worker resides, even for a short time. Even where a series of offences, for example, indecent assaults, have been apparently committed by one man breaking into ground-floor bedrooms, no liability would be imposed upon those managing the hostel or residence for failing to prevent further assaults, unless they had, perhaps, unreasonably failed to repair a broken door or window.

When a crime of violence is committed, we do not normally think of the civil obligation that the offender now owes the victim; yet every criminal offence against the person (and against property) is also a civil wrong (called a tort). Accordingly, where he or she is injured by a patient, a health-care worker should initially think of the possibility of a civil action. This will be an action for assault and battery, which, depending on the severity of the injury, will be heard in the County Court or the High Court. Provided that there are credible witnesses to give evidence of the assault (and there will need to be such witnesses if criminal proceedings are to succeed) and that the patient has sufficient funds (which, if the injury is minor, may well be the case), there is every reason to consider this possibility. Civil actions against offenders are rare, largely because victims believe, probably correctly, that their offenders, often being young or unemployed, are unlikely to have much money.

In general, victims leave to the police (and hence to the Crown Prosecution Service (CPS)) any proceedings that should be taken. Where the offence is not committed by a patient or if the offender's identity is otherwise unknown, there can clearly be no question either of civil action or of criminal proceedings. Even if the offender is apprehended and prosecuted to conviction, there is no guarantee that he or she will have sufficient funds to warrant a subsequent civil action. These considerations are relevant to the choice between what constitutes the two most realistic possibilities for health-care workers to obtain compensation for injuries arising from their becoming the victim of an offence involving personal violence. The first is that, following the conviction of the offender, the court makes a compensation order in the worker's favour, payable by the offender via a magistrates' court. Clearly, this possibility is dependent on the offender's being convicted, and upon his or her having some funds with which he or she can pay the order. Where the offender is not convicted (possibly because his or her identity was never known) or, if convicted, is without sufficient funds, the second possibility is an award made by the Criminal Injuries Compensation Board (CICB), to which it is necessary to make an application. Each possibility has its advantages and disadvantages, which will be detailed in the next two sections.

COMPENSATION ORDERS

Injuries covered

The law governing compensation orders is to be found in Sections 35–8 of the Powers of Criminal Courts Act 1973 as amended by the Criminal Justice Acts of 1982 and 1988. These permit a Crown Court or a magistrates' court to impose an order upon an offender convicted before it, requiring him to pay compensation to anyone who has sustained any personal injury, loss, or damage as a result of the offence or of one taken into consideration. Some of the advantages of the compensation order can be seen here.

First, although this chapter is principally concerned with compensation for injuries arising from personal violence, a compensation order can be made in respect not only of personal injury, but also of the loss of or damage to property. Suppose a health-care worker is robbed on the way home. Upon conviction the offender can be ordered to pay for the theft of a wallet or handbag (assuming they are not returned), for the repair of clothing or personal accoutrements torn or broken in the attack, as well as for such personal injuries as cuts or bruises sustained by the victim. Second, while the court may order the offender to pay compensation for personal injury arising from the offence, the offence itself does not have to be a crime of violence. Suppose the worker returns home to find that he or she has been burgled. There is well-substantiated research which shows that burglary victims frequently suffer shock. This arises from a combination of feelings, of having one's privacy invaded (some female victims speak of a feeling almost of being sexually compromised), of anger, of depression, and of a heightened fear of crime. There is no doubt that the court could include in the order a sum by way of compensation for this trauma.

So far as crimes of violence against the person are concerned, a compensation order can be made in respect both of physical injuries and of mental injuries, such as might arise from a straight-forward case of an offence of wounding under section 20 or assault occasioning actual bodily harm under section 47 of the Offences against the Person Act 1861. Such an event is not unusual in an A&E department on a Friday or Saturday night: cuts, scarring, broken noses and jaws, shock and distress may result. There may be some difficulty where the offender is mentally ill, as this could preclude a conviction if he or she didn't know what he or she was doing; and where the offender is elderly, the CPS may consider a prosecution inappropriate. If the injury is serious, an application to the CICB may succeed (see below). It is, however, no impediment to a conviction for these offences that the offender was voluntarily intoxicated, whether through drink or drugs. The courts take a robust view of self-induced intoxication; they treat this as reckless conduct, and it is no defence to a charge involving an offence which can be committed recklessly, that the perpetrator was so intoxicated that he or she didn't know what he or she was doing.

Compensation can also be ordered in respect of convictions for sexual offences, whether, as is typically the case in rape, they result in physical injury, or, as in indecent exposure or assault, they result primarily in shock. In any of these cases, an order may be made in favour of a victim who suffers physical or mental injury or both. A 'peeping tom' does not specifically commit a criminal offence; however, if it is his intention, for example, to frighten a nurse by peering through her bedroom window while she is undressing, he may be guilty of an offence under section 47, since 'actual bodily harm' includes occasioning in the victim an hysterical and nervous condition. It is also possible that a 'peeping tom' could commit an offence under section 5 of the Public Order Act 1986, in which case a compensation order could be made against him on conviction.

So far we have assumed that the health-care worker who has suffered the personal injury specified by section 35 of the 1973 Act is the same person as the victim of the offence for which the offender is convicted. Of course, in most cases it will be, but it need not be: the worker who suffers shock as a consequence of being a witness to an offence against another, or, perhaps, who comes upon another person who is lying unconscious having been the victim of a crime, is also covered by this section. A nurse who attends upon the victims of a terrorist bomb explosion, for example, is in theory covered, though it is no doubt unlikely that an order would be made in such a case, the offender being sent to prison for many years. Nevertheless, there is an important point here to which we shall return.

Compensation orders can also be made in respect of an offence that is taken into consideration by the court when sentencing the offender. This process is a common occurrence with minor property offences; it enables the police to treat the offences as 'cleared up', and in practice it means that the offender won't be convicted and sentenced for all of them. Thus, it may be possible for a victim of theft, of taking and driving away, or of criminal damage, to obtain compensation even though no conviction is returned. In the case of personal injury, however, this is unlikely, as a court would not be prepared to take offences of violence against the person into consideration upon sentence.

There are a number of limitations on the scope of compensation orders. They are not payable where the offender has been cautioned. Cautioning is a standard response to first-time offenders committing property offences; it is thus unlikely to affect, one way or the other, health-care workers who are the victims of crimes of violence. Injuries arising from road-traffic offences are, with one small exception, excluded. Neither can compensation be ordered in respect of loss of dependency, that is the loss of income of the deceased, occasioned by homicide. The exception here is for what is called bereavement. Suppose a murdered worker had been married; a compensation order may be made in favour of his or her spouse. The only other case allowed by law will not apply, since it relates to a case where the deceased was under 18. Where the bereavement award is payable, it is for a sum not exceeding the maximum laid down in the Fatal Accidents Act 1976, currently £7500.

Assessing the offender's means

All that has been said so far is, of course, dependent on the offender's having sufficient funds to pay compensation. Before it makes an order the court must comply with its statutory duty to take the offender's means into account. If the offender indicates a willingness to pay compensation, a court will usually take that at its face value, though it must satisfy itself about the sources from which these funds will be drawn. An offender who asserts that he's got a stash of money in a suitcase in a left-luggage locker in Paris is unlikely to have an order made against him. The problem for the court is that if it makes an order with which the offender can't comply, he is likely to return to crime so as to meet it. If he has a capital asset, a car perhaps, there is no objection to the court's making an order on the basis that he will have to sell it, provided that it can place reasonably clear value upon it. Nor is there any objection to an order's being made against an offender on income support. The Home Office has indicated that, in such circumstances, payment of £5.00 a week may be proper; this does, of course, have serious implications for the total amount that the offender may be able to pay. An unwillingness to pay should not deter the court from making an order if it is obvious that the offender has some financial resources.

A Crown Court judge can make a compensation order for any amount at all; but in the magistrates' courts, where the vast majority of orders are made, the Criminal Justice Act 1991 imposes a maximum of £5000 for any one offence (previously £2000). Within either this statutory limit or the limit imposed in practice by the amount the offender is able to pay, the order is payable as a lump sum or in instalments, usually over not more than 3 years. As we will see, the number of victims who recover under compensation orders is low, as is the amount that they recover.

Assessing the amount of compensation

On the assumption that the offender has some funds, the next step is for the court to determine how much he ought to pay the victim. This depends first on how extensive are his resources, and second on the severity of the injuries sustained. Clearly, if the offender is on income support and the victim was blinded in one eye (an injury that would attract £16 000–18 000 general damages in a civil action), the order will come nowhere close to compensating the victim. Indeed, in a case where there is a great discrepancy between what the offender can afford and the severity of the injuries, the court may well not make any order. Here we see the principal obstacle to a health-care worker's obtaining full compensation from the offender for the injuries he inflicted. If the injuries are minor, full compensation may be made, albeit in instalments; but if their value exceeds what the court thinks it proper for him to pay, the victim will only receive some of the 'ideal' value of the injuries. Of course it remains open to the worker to sue the offender. A civil court does not have to take the defendant's means into account when making its order, which could of course result in his bankruptcy; but given an offender with little resources, the health-worker may not think it worth the trouble. As we shall see, if the injuries are severe and uncompensated by the offender, the worker may succeed in an application to the CICB; but there are some limitations there.

Like the assessment of damages in a civil action, the evaluation by a criminal court of a victim's injury in respect of which it is considering making a compensation order comprises two elements: one sum to reflect general damages, that is, to include what is called pain and suffering and loss of amenities, and the second to reflect special damages, that is, to include material losses, such as loss of income and expenses.

General damages

In 1988 a set of guidelines was published indicating the figure that would be appropriate for given personal injuries, being the ones most commonly appearing before magistrates. They have not yet been officially updated, but it would be appropriate to regard them all as being index-linked. The figures are based on the likely effects of an injury of the specified kind being sustained by a person of between 20 and 35 years of age, of average health, and with no particular susceptibilities. The guidelines recommend that the age and the sex of the victim be treated as factors that may materially affect the assessment. Particular mention is made of the impact of scarring upon the victim; a scar which can be seen when the victim is fully clothed, especially if it is on the face, should normally be treated as more serious that one concealed by clothing. Generally speaking, a court will regard as more serious scarring on a woman than scarring on a man.

The figures given in Table 6.1 reflect what the law calls 'pain and suffering', that is, the normal physical and mental distress associated with the particular injury. They also include the normal 'loss of amenity' that such injury causes, for example, being unable to pursue a hobby or to engage in a sport. Where there is a particular sensitivity that aggravates the injury, or where, for example, the worker is a county standard squash player now unable to compete in a national competition, it may be possible to persuade the court to increase the amount payable; but as always, this will be subject to what the court considers the offender can be properly ordered to pay. Moreover, magistrates are unwilling to become involved in more complicated assessments of the loss to the victim. If an offender is on trial at the Crown Court, a Circuit or High Court judge will be better placed to assess general damages in such a case; but in general, if the injury requires anything other than a simple assessment (especially if the prognosis is unclear), the court will be reluctant to make an order.

Violence in health care

Table 6.1 Pain and suffering guidelines in magistrates' courts (1988)

Type of injury		Suggested award
graze	depending on size	up to £50
bruise	depending on size	up to £75
black eye		£100
cut (without permanent scarring)	depending on size and whether stitched	£75–£200
sprain	depending on loss of mobility	£100–£400
loss of a tooth (not a front tooth)	depending on position of tooth and age of victim	£250–£500
minor injury	causing reasonable absence from work of about 3 weeks	£550
loss of front tooth		£1000
facial scar	(however small) resulting in permanent disfigurement	£550+
facial scar	a vicious slash wound leaving scar from ear to corner of the mouth or under the chin	£5000–£8000
jaw	fractured (wired)	£1750
nose	undisplaced fracture of the nasal bone	£550
nose	displaced fracture of the nasal bone requiring manipulation under general anaesthetic	£850
nose	not causing fracture but displaced septum requiring a sub-mucous resection	£1500
wrist	simple fracture with complete recovery in a few weeks	£1750–£2500

Special damages

'Special damages' covers all those material losses that flow from the injury, for example, loss of earnings, the cost of dental treatment such as the repair or replacement of dentures, hearing-aids and spectacles, and expenses incurred in travelling to and from the worker's GP or to an out-patients' department. Health-care workers who have a contract of employment with a health authority or trust will usually not lose any earnings, as they will continue to be paid; on the other hand, a bank or agency nurse is usually not paid unless working. It is therefore very important that such a worker keeps a clear and accurate record of the number of days lost as a consequence of the injury. Some health-care workers who live at home also look after their elderly parents; if the consequence of the injury is that someone else has to be engaged to care for the house and/or parents, this expense too is covered by the heading 'special damages'. As ever, whether an order is made to cover this expense will depend on the offender's resources.

Whatever the material loss for which the victim is seeking compensation, the court will in every case require evidence of the loss, and may ask for receipts, pay slips, bills, and other documentary evidence of payments made or owed by the worker as a result of the injury. A victim is strongly advised to make sure that these details are kept safely. Even if there is limited success in obtaining a compensation order, these details will be needed should a claim be made to the CICB.

What you need to do

Unlike the CICB, there is no official application procedure that you need to follow for the court to consider whether it should order your offender to pay you compensation. Remember that the court is not obliged to make an order in your favour. However, the court is under a statutory duty to give reason why it hasn't made an order in a case in which it has power to do so. If you have appeared as a prosecution witness in your offender's trial, and during your evidence you told the court about the injuries he inflicted on you, the court would be acting unlawfully if it did not then give a reason why it has not, upon his conviction, ordered him to compensate you. If the reason it gives is that it has considered his means to be insufficient, then you have no ground for complaint. Likewise if it makes an order for a smaller sum than the full value of your injuries; but if it makes no order and says nothing at all, then you should seek legal advice. You are 'a person aggrieved' within section 111 of the Magistrates' Courts Act 1980, and should ask for an appeal by way of case stated to the High Court.

Another reason that the court could properly give for not making an order in your case is that it had insufficient evidence upon which to establish to its satisfaction the kind of injury you sustained and its impact upon you: your evidence that the offender ran up to you and hit you with a bottle may be quite sufficient to convict him of an offence of wounding, but it won't be sufficient to determine what amount of compensation you should be paid, even given that he is apparently well off. Even though you may be the chief prosecution witness, you have no right to speak to the court about your injuries except in answer to the questions put to you; you cannot address the court in your own right about your loss of earnings or medical expenses. Neither do you have any right to speak up at the sentencing stage, which is the time when the court will be considering the question of compensation. How then, is the court going to know about your injuries and the impact they have had on you?

The answer is to make sure that when you report the offence to the police (or if someone else reports on your behalf) that the police fill in, or let you fill in, a 'Compensation Schedule'. If you are asked to attach copies of receipts and bills, always make sure you keep your own copy. All police forces have been instructed by the Home Office to give assistance to victims of crime, and to use this Schedule, which asks for details of any injury, loss, or damage, as a means by which the court will be informed of your circumstances. The Schedule is attached to the case papers forwarded to the CPS, who should in turn notify the magistrates or the trial judge of its contents. If the police to whom you speak don't know about the Schedule, refer to the Home Office circular No. 20/1988.

An alternative is to get in touch with the national organization, Victim Support (for address and telephone number see Appendix), which is a charity specifically established to help victims of crime. Besides exploring compensation possibilities, it operates a volunteer counselling service. Victim Support has 300 branches, listed in local telephone directories. You may well find that, if your injury is serious, the local branch will get in touch with you (each one is routinely informed by the police of offences of personal violence, given of course, that the police have recorded the offence).

Success rates

While, in theory, compensation orders offer a quick and simple means by which a victim can obtain compensation from the offender, they have in the past not been much used following convictions for offences involving personal violence. However over the past three years there has been a substantial increase in the number of orders made by magistrates in such cases.

In 1991 a total of 113 000 orders were made, 107 000 by magistrates and 10 400 by the Crown Court. In the case of indictable offences of violence against the person, 19 600 orders were made by magistrates (against 58 per cent of all offenders sentenced for this type of offence) and 3500 were made by the Crown Court (25 per cent of offenders). There were 300 orders made by magistrates on conviction for robbery (on 40 per cent of offenders) and 200 at the Crown Court (5 per cent of offenders). For sexual offences, 200 orders were made following summary conviction (against 10 per cent of offenders), and 100 were made by the Crown Court (2 per cent of offenders) (*Criminal Statistics England and Wales 1991, 1993*: Table 7.24). There are a number of reasons why these figures are low, but the introduction in 1988 of both the Compensation Schedule and the guideline figures for general damages, and the imposition in 1989 of the statutory duty on a court to give reasons why it hasn't made an order when it could, does appear to have encouraged the courts to make orders in more cases. In 1988, apart from a lower total of orders for offences of violence against the person (12 600 in magistrates' courts, 3 000 in Crown Courts), the proportion of offenders ordered to pay compensation was lower in each court than in 1991 (34 per cent and 19 per cent).

No amount of Schedules, guidelines or statutory duties will make any difference if offenders are of limited means. In 1991, the average amount ordered to be paid by magistrates in the case of violence against the person was £125, and in the case of sexual offences, £105. In the Crown Court, these amounts were £318 and £295 respectively. By comparison, the highest average figure in the magistrates' court for any one offence was £225 (theft and handling) and the average for all indictable offences was £125; in the Crown Court these averages were £2981 (fraud and forgery) and £882 respectively. The figures for personal injury are very low; even if the average figure in a magistrates' court (£125) was an amount payable only in respect of pain and suffering, it is an amount commensurate with virtually the lowest figure on the Home Office's recommended tariff, payable in respect of a black eye or sprain (£100) or a minor cut (£75–£200). As it is unlikely that all 19 300 victims in whose favour orders were made in 1991 sustained only such minor injury, the primary reason for these low figures is almost certainly that in most cases the court considered that this was all the offender could afford, irrespective of the tariff value of the injury.

Around 80 per cent of offenders eventually comply with the orders made against them. Payment by instalments may well take over a year (that is, of course, after the delay in bringing the offender to trial, which may be a few weeks in the magistrates' courts, but months in the Crown Court). Despite these considerations, a health-care worker who suffers a fairly minor injury, caused by an offender with means, stands a good chance of becoming the beneficiary of a compensation order. If the injuries are severe, it is very unlikely to reflect their 'value' according to law. In this case, the only recourse is to apply to the CICB.

THE CRIMINAL INJURIES COMPENSATION SCHEME

Injuries covered

The Criminal Injuries Compensation Board (CICB) administers a non-statutory Scheme under which victims of crimes of violence may be compensated for the injuries they sustained, and where they die in consequence, under which their dependants can be compensated. The Scheme applies throughout England, Wales, and Scotland and is funded by the government, and there is therefore no question of the making of the award or of the payment of the compensation's being dependent on the offender's resources. Clearly, this is a very substantial advantage by comparison with compensation orders. So far as its scope is concerned, the Scheme differs from compensation orders in two main ways.

First, it only applies to personal injuries. With one exception to be mentioned later, no compensation can be awarded for any loss of or damage to property, or for injury arising from the commission of an offence against property. A health-care worker who is robbed can be compensated for the physical and mental injury that is caused, but not for the loss of or damage to possessions. There can, however, be no compensation for the shock of discovering that one has been burgled, no matter how great the burglary or the shock, because burglary is a crime against property. The kinds of injury that constitute 95 per cent of the claims that the CICB receives arise from offences such as assault occasioning actual bodily harm, wounding, and causing grievous bodily harm under sections 47, 20, and 18 respectively of the Offences against the Person Act 1861. Depending on the severity of the injury, and whether it was recklessly or intentionally inflicted, this part of the Scheme covers, for example, nurses and porters injured by drunks in an A&E department on a Friday and Saturday night, robberies, or other violent assaults. The Scheme will also cover the offences of rape and indecent assault. Indecent exposure is not a crime of violence but maybe covered by paragraph 10. There are four other circumstances in which a health-care worker may sustain an injury, whether on or off duty, that are covered by this Scheme.

(a) Injuries arising from arson; this covers the worker who, while attending at the scene a person burnt or overcome by fumes in an arson attack on a building, is injured by the collapse of a part of the building, or is overcome by fumes.

(b) Injuries caused by an offence of poisoning. This does not cover accidental or negligent poisoning.

(c) Injuries arising from trespass on a railway. This was introduced to bring within the scope of the Scheme railway employees who suffer shock either from witnessing people committing suicide under their own trains, or from dealing with the corpse of a suicide. The health-worker who suffers shock in consequence of witnessing either of these events would likewise come within the Scheme.

(d) Injuries arising from efforts by the victim to enforce the law, perhaps by giving help to a policeman. Suppose a nurse tries to sedate the violent offender a policeman is endeavouring to restrain, and is injured by a weapon held in the offender's flailing hands. The nurse who could show that the offender intentionally or recklessly inflicted the injury would clearly come within the scope of the Scheme's main provision, namely, that injury was caused by the commission of a crime of violence. If, however, the injury was sustained accidently (being now sedated, the offender falls against the nurse) or as a result of the offender's negligence (now wishing to give himself up, he throws the weapon to one side, where it strikes the nurse), he or she would not be the victim of a crime of violence. However, the nurse who was taking an exceptional risk in helping the policeman will come within the Scheme. What is an exceptional risk will depend upon the circumstances, but for a private citizen to assist in the restraint of an armed offender would probably be so regarded.

In all these instances, like a compensation order, the Scheme permits compensation to be awarded where the health-care worker suffers physical injury only, mental injury only, or both. Also like a compensation order, the Scheme permits compensation to be awarded where the worker suffers shock from witnessing an attack on another, or the aftermath of an attack on another. For example, a nurse who suffers shock from dealing with the victims of a terrorist bomb explosion is in theory compensatable by means of a compensation order should the offenders be convicted, but this is unlikely to happen in practice because the offender's means will probably be inadequate. However, under the Scheme, there would be no difficulty, as the offender's position is irrelevant.

The second main difference is that there is no requirement for an award of compensation under the Scheme that there be a conviction against the offender (though this will help), or even that the offender be identified. This is obviously of great importance where the worker is attacked by someone who is not a patient. It is also of importance where the worker is attacked by a patient against whom, because of his mental condition, criminal proceedings are unlikely to be taken or to succeed. The Board's approach in such cases is to ask whether, had the assailant been in command of his faculties, he would have appreciated what he was doing.

There is one exception to the absence of any requirement of the identification of the assailant: if the victim is injured by someone with whom he or she is living (parent, lover, or other), then there must be good reasons why the offender has not been prosecuted. The victim will also have to show, in the case of violence within the family, that he or she no longer lives in the same household, and in every case, that the offender is not likely to benefit from the award.

Although, in the usual case, there need be no identification of the offender, it is vital that the health-care worker should report the incident giving rise to the injury to the police without delay. Where the offence takes place while the worker is on duty, it is quite likely that it will be reported to the police by the hospital management. This will not do for the purpose of obtaining compensation from the CICB. The Scheme is explicit: **the worker him- or herself must report the incident.**

As has been indicated, the Scheme also applies to cases in which the worker is killed in the assault; the various points made above apply equally here, with appropriate adjustments. The Scheme does not apply to injuries or fatalities arising from traffic accidents, unless the accident was a result of a deliberate attempt to hit the victim.

Eligibility for compensation

At the expense of repetition (but it is important) the first requirement is that the health-care worker him- or herself reports the incident to the police without delay. Thereafter the worker must co-operate with them in their enquiries. If the police wish to hold an identification parade, he or she must attend; fear of reprisal will not be an acceptable excuse. It is not necessary to press charges, but if the Crown Prosecution Service do, the worker must be willing, if called upon, to give evidence at the trial. The worker must also co-operate with the CICB after making the claim for compensation; withholding evidence of injury, for example, for fear of embarrassment will not be acceptable.

The claim for compensation must be made within 3 years of the incident. It is sometimes the case that many years pass before an injury's effects become evident; the Board has a discretion to allow claims made out of time, but the circumstances of the claim will be closely scrutinized.

Third, there is a minimum loss provision in the Scheme. The injury has to be 'worth' more than £1000 after any deductions the Board must make for the value of any social security benefits to which the claimant is entitled (before January 1992 this figure was £750). How does this work? As we shall see in the following section, the CICB, like magistrates' courts, have a set of guideline figures for specimen injuries. If the victim's jaw was broken in an assault, and needed an operation to be put right, the general damages award would be in the region of £2500; so without taking into account any special damages, he or she would be well over the minimum. On the other hand, an undisplaced fracture of the nose attracts a guideline figure of £650, so only if the special damages exceed £350 (and then only if there is no entitlement to social security benefits whose total would bring the total back under £1000) will the claim be considered. The minimum loss figure doesn't mean, however, that the Board won't make awards of less than £1000. If an injury is 'worth' £1100, and the victim has received the average figure from the offender under a compensation order (£114), the Board will have to take that into account, but will make an award of £986. Nevertheless, the minimum loss provision is one of the principal disadvantages of the Scheme by comparison with a compensation order; it doesn't assist victims with less serious injuries.

The final condition of eligibility concerns the victim's own behaviour. The Scheme provides that the Board may disqualify from compensation a claimant who has a conviction for a serious offence, but as such a history would in any event preclude someone from becoming a health-care worker in the first place, this can be set aside. However, the Scheme also provides that the Board may disqualify a claimant from compensation because of his or her conduct before, during, or after the events giving rise to the claim, or because of his or her unlawful conduct. If the worker provoked the assault, or was intoxicated (whether through drink or illicit drugs), and certainly if he or she struck the first blow, the Board could well refuse any or all of the claim.

Assessing the amount of compensation*

Like compensation orders, a CICB award includes both general damages and special damages; unlike them, the amount to which the victim will be entitled will always reflect (leaving aside any reduction for bad behaviour) the full value of the injury and its consequences, less any deductions for moneys received from other sources (see below). One important power that the Board has is to make further payments of compensation should the victim's condition deteriorate beyond the limits of a normal progression

---

* The Government propose to replace this system with a tariff comprising 25 monetary levels covering 186 designated injuries, from £1000 (*eg.* deviated nasal septum) to £250 000 (*eg* quadriplegia): *Compensating Victims of Violent Crime* (HMSO, 1993, Cm 2434).

Table 6.2 Guidelines for pain and suffering awards in the CICB (1991)

Injury	Suggested award
undisplaced nasal fracture	£650
displaced nasal fracture	£1000
loss of two front teeth (necessitating denture or bridge)	£1500
elevated zygoma (following injury to cheekbone)	£1500
fractured jaw (requiring an operation)	£2500
simple fracture to the tibia, fibula, ulna, or radius, with complete recovery	£2500
laparotomy (exploratory abdominal operation and scar)	£3000
scar, young man, from joint of lobe of the left ear and face across cheek within an inch of left corner of mouth	£6000
total loss of hearing (one ear)	£11 500
total loss of taste and smell as a result of a fractured skull	£12 000
total loss of vision (one eye)	£15 000

of the injury. In this respect the CICB is unlike a civil action or a compensation order, which result in once-and-for-all payments.

General damages

Where the victim survives the attack, compensation will be awarded for pain and suffering and loss of amenity, and where the injury has reduced the victim's life expectancy, for that too. The Board regularly publishes guideline figures for pain and suffering as part of its continuing efforts to ensure that its awards are in line with common law damages. Its latest figures (1991) are set out in Table 6.2.

It can be seen that no figure is given for rape. In its 1987 guidelines, the Board indicated a figure of £5000, but, in part because the Board was constantly being criticized for not placing a sufficient value on the pain of rape to a woman, it concluded that it would now be unrealistic to give any figure.

These figures are guideline figures only. They do not, and cannot, displace the Board's discretion under the Scheme to assess the compensation appropriate to each case. As with the guidelines for magistrates, in each case the figure is a starting-point, and may be increased or decreased according to circumstances. If the effect on the claimant is greater than that which such an injury usually causes, a higher award will be made. For example, many people with broken noses recover completely, but if there is any significant permanent disability or cosmetic defect, the award will be more, and perhaps substantially more, than the guideline figure. The Board is also conscious of the differential impact on male and female victims of scarring, and the corresponding variations in the award will be made. Likewise an elderly victim sustaining a minor assault may well be made an award higher than would be made if the victim were young. Women will also note that the Board is prepared to increase awards (for example for rape) because of the woman's fear that she may develop AIDS. This could apply also if a health-care worker were injured by a hypodermic needle used by an HIV-positive offender, or contracted hepatitis B as a result of an assault with a needle.

In cases where the victim is unlawfully killed, and the dependants (spouse, parents, grandparents, or children) are the claimants, the only general damages that may be awarded are the same as apply to civil actions: the bereavement award. Unlike compensation orders, where the sum payable may not exceed the statutory maximum, the award will be for the full amount, currently £7500.

Special damages

With one exception, compensation is payable under the Scheme only for personal injuries. An award in respect of the loss of or damage to property may be made if the Board is satisfied that it was relied upon by the victim as a physical aid. This primarily covers personal items ('adjuncts') such as spectacles, dentures, hearing-aids, and artificial limbs. No compensation will be awarded for jewellery, watches, or rings lost or damaged at the time of or after the incident, or in the course of medical or other treatment arising therefrom. Nor will an award be made in respect of lost or damaged clothing. Where an award is made in respect of personal adjuncts, it will only be for such amount as is necessary to render them usable, or to replace them with a pair of equal utility.

On the assumption that the health-care worker can verify each item, the Board will routinely include in the award compensation for medical and other expenses, for example, dental costs, fares to hospitals, and the cost of any treatment prescribed. Where the injuries sustained require long-term care for the victim, including, for example, alterations to the victim's house or domestic arrangements where he or she has been disabled by the injury, expenses incurred will be compensatable as at common law. The Board's Reports show awards covering the cost of rehabilitation courses; blind aids, talking watches, and home assistance for victims blinded by an attack; for nursing care; for changes to the structure and layout of a house, including the provision of additional heating; and for the provision of an adapted car for victims handicapped by paralysis. The Board will endeavour to make provision for any increases in such expenses that are now foreseeable. Expenses or losses incurred by others, for example, the loss of present or future income earned by a spouse or parent who gives up a job to nurse the victim, are compensatable.

It is assumed that the medical treatment sought by, and provided to, the victim will be provided by the NHS. The cost of private medical treatment will be payable by the Board only if it considers that, in all the circumstances, both the private treatment and the cost of it are reasonable. What is 'reasonable' is a matter of opinion, but it would probably cover a young woman who would otherwise have to wait for many months or even years for plastic surgery to correct the facial scars left by the criminal injury.

Pain and suffering experienced by a rape victim is compensatable, as is any pain and suffering associated with any consequent pregnancy and any expenses associated with any consequent birth. The Scheme does not, however, permit compensation to be paid for the maintenance of the child; what is provided is an additional sum, currently £5000, payable to each child born and conceived as a result of the rape which the mother, at the time of the award, intends to keep. This sum is not recoverable by the Board should she later seek to have the child adopted.

Legal costs incurred by the claimant in the preparation of an application to the Board are not compensatable. Neither will the Board reimburse a claimant for the costs incurred in pursuing an unsatisfied judgement in civil proceedings.

The victim is entitled to damages for loss of earnings to the date of the trial and for future loss of earnings. Loss of earnings can generally be calculated by reference to wage or salary slips. Here again, if the worker has a contract of employment, he or she is unlikely to lose any earnings, at least in the short term. Agency and bank nurses should make sure they keep an account of how much income they have lost while unable to work. There is a limit on how much compensation a victim will receive under the Scheme: it shall not exceed twice the gross average industrial earnings at the date of assessment (an upper limit which would currently amount to around £20 000 a year).

In cases where the victim is unlawfully killed, those dependants who can show a loss of dependency are eligible for compensation: for example, an elderly parent supported by a son or daughter, a child supported by its parent, or a spouse. It is important to stress that there has to be a measurable loss of income to the dependant to qualify under this heading. If there is none, the only compensation is for bereavement, and that is quite narrowly confined.

Deductions

From any award of compensation that the CICB makes must be deducted the full value of virtually every other sum of money that the claimant receives in consequence of the injury. The main exception is that sums accruing from personally effected insurance policies (which includes policies subscribed to by a claimant's parents when he or she was under 18) are excluded. So too are awards for bravery or from a charitable source. Otherwise, the value of all social security benefits, occupational pensions, employer's insurance and sick pay is fully deductible from the award; not just from the element of special damage, but from the global sum. In other words, if the amount of such benefits to be deducted exceeds the amount of special damages payable under the Scheme, the balance will be deducted from the element of general damages.

In addition, any moneys received from the offender by way of a compensation order will be deducted from the award. When the Board notifies you of the award, you are required to confirm that you will in turn pay over any such moneys you may receive.

What you need to do

To obtain an application form write to:

Criminal Injuries Compensation Authority
Tay House
300 Bath Street
GLASGOW G2 4JR

It is also possible that your local police station may have forms. If you have trouble filling them in, ask for help from your local branch of Victim Support, or write to them in London if there is no branch near you (see Appendix for details).

Before you send your completed form, make a copy. Your claim will be dealt with initially by letter. The Board will certainly seek to verify what you have said by writing to the police, your employer, and those who have given you medical treatment. They may also write to you for clarification of matters raised by your claim. Do not be tempted to exaggerate your injuries; give as succinct and accurate an account of their impact as you can. You will in due course receive a letter giving the Board's determination of your claim. You may accept it; but you also have the right to question it. Be careful! If you question a low award, you suspend any entitlement you would otherwise have to it; in other words, if on appeal the Board thinks its original 'low' award was too high, it is free to reduce it further, and you will have no remedy. Consult a lawyer if you wish to question the Board's decision. If you question the Board's initial determination, you may have the opportunity to argue your claim at an oral hearing, but not in all cases. Here too, it may help if you can elicit the support of your union or professional body, or a solicitor (but not one who asks for a cut from any compensation you should be awarded).

Success rates

In 1991/92 the Board received 61 400 claims for compensation. Although there is no direct correlation between these figures, in the same year it resolved 60 113 claims, paying out £128 529 159. Over the lifetime of the Board, about 60–65 per cent of claimants have been successful. The sums awarded can be substantial, following the common law's valuation of injuries; the majority (68 per cent) receive more than £1000 (Criminal Injuries Compensation Board, 1992; paras. 1.2, 8.2).

Unquestionably one of the most frustrating features of the CICB is the time it takes to resolve claims for compensation. Seventy per cent of claims take more than 9 months to resolve; 55 per cent take more than 12 months. There is little you can do about this, even if your claim is straightforward. Be prepared for a long wait!

SUMMARY

1. If the injury you have sustained is fairly minor (as most are) – bruising; cuts requiring a few stitches; a broken tooth; wrist, neck or shoulder sprain; or a small scar – and your offender is to be prosecuted for an offence which caused it, try for a compensation order.

2. If you do, make sure you fill in or get the police to fill in a Compensation Schedule. Keep a record of any costs, including loss of earnings, that you have incurred as a result of the injury. Keep copies.

3. Make a note of the name of the police officer who deals with your claim, and of his/her station phone number.

4. If you are not called as a prosecution witness, pester your local Crown Prosecution Service (make a note of their telephone number) to tell you the date of the trial. If your offender is convicted, and he is remanded for sentencing, pester them to tell you when the sentencing hearing will be. That's when the question of compensation will arise.

5. Don't have great expectations of large sums by way of compensation. The average figure ordered by magistrates in 1990 for offences of wounding and occasioning actual bodily harm was £114. If your offender really is penniless, you probably won't get anything.

6. If your injury is complex, or its prognosis unclear, it is likely that the court won't make an order.

7. If the injury you have sustained involves at least scarring (especially to the face), a broken arm, leg, rib, jaw, or nose, or the loss of more than one tooth, you should certainly make a claim to the CICB.

8. If you do, you MUST *personally* report the incident to the police without delay.

9. Write to the CICB in Glasgow for a claim form. Keep a copy of the completed form that you return. Keep a record of any costs, including loss of earnings, that you have incurred as a result of the injury. Also keep a note of any sick pay or other payments you receive in consequence of the injury.

10. Take legal advice before questioning the Board's initial determination.

11. You will see that there are two groups of victims who are likely to fall between these two remedies:
    (a) those victims whose offenders were convicted but against whom a compensation order was not made, or was made in an amount less than the value of the injuries they sustained, if those injuries are worth less than £1000; and
    (b) those victims whose offenders were not convicted and whose injuries are worth less than £1000.
       Sad to say, there is no practical hope for compensation in either case. The irony is that if a victim's offender is neither convicted nor worth pursuing through either the criminal or the civil courts, the health-care worker's best chance of compensation is if she or he is caused more harm than the CICB's minimum loss requirement.

12. If you need some practical help, get in touch with your local branch of Victim Support.

FURTHER READING

Criminal Injuries Compensation Board (1992). *Twenty-eighth Report*, Cm 2122. HMSO, London.

Donnelly, C. (1991). Ending the torment. *Nursing Times*, **87**, 36–8.

Miers, D. (1990). *Compensation for criminal injuries*. Butterworth, London.

Shepherd, J. (1990). Violent Crime in Bristol. *British Journal of Criminology*, **30**, 289–305.

Whittington, R. and Wykes, T. (1989). Invisible injury. *Nursing Times*, **85**, 30–2.

7 Domestic violence

John Gayford

The study of domestic violence only began in the 1970s, which is surprising, as in retrospect there is plenty of evidence of domestic violence in history. As is the case with child abuse, it was more comfortable for professional health workers to accept explanations offered to cover up the real cause of the injuries, and it is only in the last two decades that the full horror of the problem has gradually been revealed.

DEFINITION OF DOMESTIC VIOLENCE

Strictly speaking, domestic violence is violence which occurs within the home, between people who have a close relationship. In this sense it would be seen to be the same as family violence, and includes:

1. Violence between husband and wife (this would include those in cohabitation).
2. Violence between parent and children (this would include incidents where the child is the victim, but would also include incidents where the parent, usually in his or her declining years, is the victim).
3. Violence between people living in a homosexual relationship.

In this chapter the emphasis will be on violence between husbands and wives, and violence is taken to mean the use of physical force which has resulted in demonstrable physical injury. Some would see this as a narrow definition, and would quite rightly point to the even more long-term damage and suffering which can result from repeated psychological cruelty and degradation, to the point where the victim loses all self-respect and dignity. Many sad cases are known where the victims are driven to inflicting damage on themselves by means of self-mutilation and drug abuse, and even the ultimate self-abuse of suicide.

Battered wife

This was a deliberatively emotive term introduced by Erin Pizzey in 1971 in her book *Scream quietly or the neighbours will hear* to draw attention to women who were the victims of serious domestic violence. The Royal College of Psychiatrists persisted with the term. The use of the word 'battered' implies that repeated blows have been struck, usually by a man losing control. The following definition is well established:

'Any woman who has received deliberate, severe, repeated, demonstrable physical injury from her marital partner'.

Marital partners include both spouses and those in a cohabitation; but most surveys exclude injuries received by women who were in a courting relationship, but not actually living with a partner. As about 25 per cent of battered wives are subjected to violence in the courting period, this definition does not include all non-accidental injuries to women.

It is clear that this definition pays no heed to psychological cruelty on its own. This can have equally profound effects, not only on the victim herself, but also on any children of the relationship, and, as with physical violence, can become a learned pattern of behaviour which may continue into the next generation.

Marital or conjugal violence

This term has the advantage of not defining the sex of either the aggressor or the victim. Nevertheless there is general agreement that in the majority of cases the woman is the victim and the man the aggressor. Even allowing for gross under-reporting in criminal statistics, three-quarters of the victims are female. In one study over 97 per cent of the offenders were male and over 94 per cent of the victims were female. Even in such extreme cases as when a woman has used a weapon to kill her husband, there is often a long history of her having been subjected to repeated physical violence over a considerable period of time.

Tortured wife

In 1878 Cobbe used this highly emotive term to sensationalize her argument when trying to make her point to an unsympathetic Victorian society. If this term is to be used, it is best to reserve it for the fortunately very rare cases in which a woman is subjected to calculated sadistic attacks.

Spouse abuse

This is the term preferred by many authors, as it widens the definition to include psychological abuse, and does not define the sex of either the aggressor or the victim. This is a pattern of behaviour in a relationship in which one person victimizes the other. The abuse may be physical, sexual, verbal, or even psychological. This term can refer to the intensive and continuous degradation and intimidation which is used for the purpose of controlling the actions or behaviour of the other person, or for placing that other person in fear of serious bodily injury, whether to the self or to others.

CAUSE AND BACKGROUND

There is little doubt that violence breeds violence. About a quarter of battered wives have actually witnessed their fathers' violence towards their mothers. This violence had extended to the woman herself, mostly from the father and sometimes from the mother.

Men who abuse their wives are even more likely to have come from violent families and to have been subjected to violence themselves. In one study, of men who battered their wives, only 38 per cent had not witnessed violence between their parents.

The effect this has on children in terms of their behavioural functioning can be dramatic, and includes temper tantrums, conduct disorder, over-sensitivity, attention problems, and anxiety withdrawal. Again, children from violent families perform less well than do those from non-violent families in terms of learning abilities at school. When it comes to emotional functioning, these children are handicapped by the multiple traumatic events they have witnessed. Later in life they have a higher risk of developing what are called somatization disorders; symptoms are produced for which there is no underlying physical cause, and about which there are multiple complaints requiring medical attention. These speculations seem to be valid, but need further scientific evaluation before they can be taken for granted (see Chapter 9).

Men, it is claimed, have used superior physical strength to maintain their dominance of the family. If the head of the family feels his authority is being threatened, then violence is the ultimate way of restoring it. This is a learned pattern of behaviour passed on from generation to generation and consciously used by some men, at whose level of sensitivity it seems to work, at least at first. If a wife threatens a domineering husband who has been brought up in this way, then violence is always possible. Some men have to act in this way as they do not possess the inner strength of character to get their way by more subtle means. They are not able to accept a challenge to their authority, nor can they accept that they are wrong. Such acceptances or admissions are seen as a threat to their self-esteem, and the only way they can see of dealing with this is by violence.

SOCIOLOGICAL FACTORS

Domestic violence has traditionally been associated with the lower social classes. This view may be challenged by the claim that the higher social classes are better at concealing their domestic violence, and do not have to resort to public support agencies when it does occur. Poor housing, poverty, and overcrowding are frustrating and stress-provoking factors which can predispose to marital violence in families in which there are other factors which make violence a likely pattern of behaviour (see Chapter 9).

It might be assumed that education would be a protective factor against family violence; but some of the women seen at refuges for battered wives have high levels of education (in terms of examination results). On the surface, one would think these women would be capable of dealing with the crises in their lives; but with a greater realization of the stress the violent crisis creates, it is appreciated that they suffer from a form of post-traumatic stress disorder which robs them of their normal coping abilities. Thus they are drawn into this helpless victim syndrome, upon which is superimposed their physical injuries.

Social isolation may also be an aetiological factor. There is no doubt that extended family support is an important preventive factor, and that other family members will sort out the problems when violence has occurred. In extreme cases they can rescue the victim from the violence and provide a refuge. The problems occur when the family are immigrants, or have moved from another part of the country. Alternatively, family relationships may be so poor that help is not sought, and in other cases the victims' families do not have the coping strengths to help, or are frightened, or may be threatened themselves by the violent man. There are even cases where male domination and violence are accepted as being normal patterns of married life.

There are no simple social explanations – only a series of complex interactions. A woman with a higher verbal capability than her husband may be the victim of his violence, which he uses as a means of asserting himself. On the other hand, a woman of low verbal ability may not be able to express and discuss her problems, and this may lead to an exacerbation of the problem and to her being subjected to his violence.

PSYCHIATRIC CAUSES AND EFFECTS OF MARITAL VIOLENCE

In the case of both the victims and the aggressors it is very difficult to differentiate between cause and effect in psychiatric conditions associated with marital violence.

Psychiatric disorders seen in battered wives

Almost half the battered women seen in one study had at some time been investigated for psychiatric problems. It is hoped that with a greater understanding of the problem there will now be less psychiatric referral and investigation, but instead, more appropriate and practical support. Anxiety and depression are common. In retrospect this is predictable, both in terms of the women and their backgrounds and the physical and psychological trauma they experience. As many women do not reveal their real problems to their general practitioners or psychiatrists, they are treated with antidepressants and tranquillizers. Those who disclose the real problem, or have it disclosed for them, often meet with a professional who has no means of helping them and who is sucked into the general frustration. In consequence they are often merely treated for the anxiety and depression. Almost three-quarters of the women in one study (70 per cent) were being prescribed tranquillizers and antidepressants. Regrettably, but again in retrospect not surprisingly, 40 per cent of the women used tablets as a means of making a suicide attempt. Most of those who had attempted suicide admitted this was a desperate bid to draw attention to their plight. They felt that if they died it would be an end to the problem, but if they lived, then something might be done for them. Many failed to provoke any positive response, and it is alarming to hear of women who have received no medical aid, but were left at home to sleep off the effects of the drugs.

Interspersed with this group are those who are prepared to indulge in substance-abuse, ranging from cannabis, through the barbiturates and benzodiazepines, to amphetamines, lysergic acid, and, in some cases, opiate alkaloids.

There is now greater awareness of the possibility of sexual abuse in childhood in any problematic group, be they alcoholics, drug-abusers, or even those with appetite disorders; and in any contemporary investigations these possibilities have to be investigated with great delicacy. Specific questions of this type were not asked in research in the early 1970s; but, even so, about 25 per cent of battered women described sexual abuse in their childhood or adolescence. Sexual abuse in childhood increases the likelihood of psychiatric disorders to about 20 per cent.

Marital rape is also a problem which is now well recognized. Some women are forced into sexual relations in the realization that refusal leads to further physical abuse, to say nothing of psychological harrassment. Some women have reported that their marital partner forced sexual relations using a weapon, such as a knife, a broken bottle, or a razor. Rough and distasteful sexual approaches are more common; many women report that their clothes had been torn off before sexual intercourse was forced upon them.

PSYCHIATRIC DISORDERS AMONG MEN VIOLENT WITHIN THE FAMILY

In studies which have been conducted into psychiatric disorders among men who are violent within the family, only alcoholism and morbid jealousy have been studied in detail; these will be described separately. Personality disorder has been much speculated upon. Other studies are far more fragmentary, and often the information obtained is indirect – for example, from women separated from their husbands while in a hostel. Husbands are frequently described by their wives as being 'schizophrenic' a favourite label used by women to indicate that the husband has two different personalities, and can change suddenly from a likeable, generous, and quite appealing person into a violent and frightening man who appears to have no control over himself. A 'Jekyll and Hyde' personality is also a term frequently used. Few cases give grounds for suspecting true schizophrenia; but many attempts have been made to explain events with a psychiatric diagnosis.

There is no doubt that the break-up of a relationship due to violence is a traumatic event for men, as well as for the women concerned. Suicide attempts are common in these circumstances, and successful suicides have been recorded. It is clear that many men develop depressive symptoms, some presenting as sad, depressed individuals, while others try to cover their symptoms with heavy drinking and aggressive, antisocial behaviour.

It is not uncommon for the combination of depression and anger to lead to self-mutilation or violent self-destructive acts. Seen from the less sympathetic viewpoint of a separated wife, these depressive, suicidal, self-destructive acts on the part of her husband are often regarded as manipulative, and as being an attempt to bring about a reconciliation by appealing to her sympathies. This may be substantiated with reports of how this has been tried before, and supported by claims that the suicide attempt was not genuine, or may even have been a lie. There is little doubt that many violent men are anxious, and try to cover their anxiety in a variety of ways. Some adopt macho façades; but in a number of cases this falls away quickly, leaving a vulnerable, dependent man as he advances in years; and indeed, a dependence on women is frequently seen in men who are violent to their wives.

PERSONALITY PROBLEMS AMONG MEN WHO ABUSE THEIR WIVES

From the treatment point of view, it is important to decide if the violence is part of a personality disorder, or is due to a psychiatric condition. The issue is further complicated by the fact that a psychiatric disorder or a personality disorder in the woman may also be an aetiological factor.

A personality disorder is 'a deeply ingrained maladaptive pattern of behaviour'. Marital violence clearly fits this description.

Not all personality disorders give rise to violence. Narcissistic, antisocial, passive-aggressive, compulsive, schizoid, and borderline personality disorders have features which can lead to violence. 'Explosive personality' is included in some classifications; but others would include this under episodic dyscontrol syndrome, which is not classified as a personality disorder. Paranoid personalities often merge into morbid jealousy with violent features. Under this heading appears the sadistic personality disorder, which fits the description given by many women of the men who are repeatedly violent to them.

Clearly, there is no one specific type of man that is responsible for domestic violence. Attempts have been made by psychologists to clarify the characteristics of men involved in family violence, and this has resulted in three sub-groups,

1   schizoid/borderline;
2   narcissistic/antisocial; and
3   dependent/compulsive.

JEALOUSY

There is little doubt that jealousy is an important factor in marital violence. In about two-thirds of cases a jealous relationship has been described, usually with pathological or morbid features. In one study one fifth of men just accused their wives of flirtatious behaviour, while one third made accusations of actual infidelity. In addition, 1 in 10 went so far as to check on their partners' activities, sometimes using the children, friends, or other relatives as agents. More rarely, professional detective agencies were used. It was not unusual for a man to want his wife or cohabitee to submit to some form of lie test. Most women were subjected to an interrogation which could last for many hours. Fortunately, cases in which the woman had been subjected to torture were rare, but when this had occurred the accounts were horrifying. Victims had their arms or fingers bent beyond the limits of extension of the joint, and cigarette lighters were used to burn the face, arms, and, in one case, the breast, and even if there was no visible injury, threats of this type were made. Four per cent of men claimed they had not sired one of the children born during the relationship.

There is a strong link between jealousy and violence. Even murder committed by men who were morbidly jealous of their female partners has been described. The seriousness of this as a complication of marital violence is thus revealed; and it indicates that immediate action needs to be taken to separate the couple while the case is investigated and before serious harm occurs.

An example of the way in which morbid jealousy complicates marital violence, or even precipitates it, is revealed in the case of a 30-year-old woman, married to a 29-year-old roofing contractor who drank heavily. Violence was usually associated with his drinking; and the fact that he had been arrested for drunken assault on the police, following an incident in which he was involved at a pub, showed that he was also violent outside the home. The couple had been married for ten years, not all of which had been violent; but violence was a common feature of the last four years of the relationship. Injuries included multiple blows to the face, with frequent bruising; and the wife also reported defective vision in one eye from a detached retina. Her nose had been fractured, and one of the upper incisor teeth had been extracted after, she claimed, it was broken by a blow. She claimed that her arms, legs, breasts, and abdomen had been bruised by punching and kicking. There was a small scar on her neck which she claimed was a stab wound from a knife. Jealousy was certainly a feature of the relationship, and had become progressively worse. She was accused of flirting and of having extramarital sexual relations, both of which she denied. Her husband frequently checked on her movements, and would check with other people to confirm her story. When she eventually refused sexual relations this was at first taken as proof of an extramarital affair; but finally she was accused of lesbianism when it was proved that she was with her female friends and not in male company.

It is not uncommon to hear of cases where a woman has left her husband and moved away. Clearly he often makes considerable efforts to trace her, and in one case a man had even gone to the lengths of finding accommodation in the road in which his wife was now living, so that he could keep her under surveillance. One older woman had repeatedly tried to leave her husband, but she claimed he would always track her down and make life so uncomfortable for her that she eventually went back to him. She claimed that on balance living with him and submitting to his dictates was preferable to constantly trying to evade him, and indeed that her absence only made him more angry and dangerous.

Cases complicated by jealousy are very time-consuming to deal with; to begin with, obtaining an accurate history is almost impossible, as both parties give radically different accounts of events and it is difficult, if not impossible, to establish the truth. Frequently there are marked personality differences between the parties: she is often easier to talk to, with a more outgoing personality, while he is usually more introverted and less articulate. In addition, he may have suspicious, obsessional features, with the result that he relates his history with an attention to detail which demands total concentration.

If treatment is to be considered, it is essential to decide whether the jealousy has any validity, or is largely delusional in nature. Morbid jealousy has been described as a multidimensional emotional state related to the unfounded suspicion of sexual and emotional rivals and a fear of losing the partner and the relationship. This manifests in behavioural disturbances. Basically, jealousy can be classified as 'normal jealousy', where there is a clear reason for the jealousy, such as the proven infidelity of the partner, and 'morbid jealousy', where the suspicion is unfounded. The problem is to define which is which and to take the appropriate action.

Alcoholism has always been seen as a major cause of morbid jealousy; and this is certainly the case in marital violence. Not only does the man's heavy drinking distort the relationship, but it affects his sexual abilities, making him a less desirable lover, particularly if the relationship has been affected by violence. Add to this a suspicious personality, and the climate is right for the growth of morbid jealousy.

Syndromes such as dementia and cerebral degeneration are possible causes, but are rarely seen in the marriages of the young. It is worth noting that morbid jealousy was found in 5 of 17 brain-damaged ex-boxers in one study, and again heavy drinking was a complicating factor. Drug abuse, particularly of substances such as cocaine and the amphetamines, and especially where persistently used, can produce a paranoid psychosis which may manifest as morbid jealousy.

In a series of cases of morbid jealousy drawn from the Maudsley Hospital, Shepherd (1961) found that the majority were suffering from paranoid schizophrenia. From a psychiatric perspective this is always a possibility that has to be considered. In the case of marital violence there is as yet little evidence of true schizophrenia in violent males.

About half of morbidly jealous people also suffer from depression. It is difficult to know whether the depression gives rise to the jealousy, or if the crisis created by the jealousy induces the depression. Once again, heavy drinking complicates the situation, as most alcoholics, seen in a crisis, have depressive symptoms.

There is a strong case for considering sexual dysfunction and obsessional neurosis as causes of morbid jealousy. Both are seen in cases of marital violence, and it is claimed that both are learned patterns of behaviour which can be treated.

Finally, there can be little doubt that personality plays an important part in the cause of morbid jealousy. The difference in personality types in the morbidly jealous relationship has already been discussed. A paranoid personality is fertile ground for the growth of morbid jealousy. In this the sufferer has a tendency to feel exploited, questions loyalty, sees threats where none exist, bears grudges, is easily slighted, and is quick to react with anger and counter-attack. One of the criteria is that they question, without justification, the fidelity of spouse or sexual partner. Once more, add alcohol to these ingredients and an explosion can be predicted.

Morbid jealousy has been considered at length because it is a dangerous complication – and some would claim a treatable disorder. It is a sign which should not be ignored, and is an indication that emergency action needs to be taken. There is a lot of truth in the old advice that the only treatment for morbid jealousy is 'a liberal dose of geography distributed between the parties'.

THE ROLE OF ALCOHOL IN MARITAL VIOLENCE

In a survey of 100 battered wives, male drunkenness was identified as the chief cause. Fifty-two per cent of men were getting drunk on a weekly basis, and another 22 per cent on a monthly basis; in 44 per cent of cases drunkenness was cited as the factor which precipitated the violence, and frequently there was some form of amnesia of the event.

It has been suggested that men drink heavily in order to give themselves an excuse to be violent to their wives. A more acceptable view would be that alcohol removes their inhibitions and allows their hostility towards their wives to be translated into violence.

Again it is clear that battered wives are not the only group of female victims resulting from male drunkenness; about two-thirds of rapists are under the influence of alcohol or drugs at the time of committing the offence. In the context of marital violence it is clear that, under the influence of alcohol, men with a propensity for violence are also likely to demand sexual relations against their partners' wishes in the same violent way. This may even follow other physical violence. In a crude way, he may in his alcoholic state see this as a way of returning the relationship to normal. Nowadays, however, this is seen as marital rape.

The effects of alcohol on marital violence have been classified in three groups: one in which alcoholism in the husband is the primary problem and the violence is related to his drinking (possibly following a row over this drinking), and a second group in which violence occurs between the couple when they have been drinking; when neither are alcoholic, nor are violent under normal circumstances. In the third, most violent group, there is a strong history of family violence. The men in this group are violent to both wives and children, with the wives reciprocating; and the highest incidence of sexual violence is found in this group. Alcoholism is not seen as the primary problem; but there is poor impulse control, both in terms of excessive drinking and of violence.

There is evidence that a smaller percentage of female victims of marital violence also drink heavily, or have drinking problems. Although women are not as likely as men to become violent under the influence of alcohol, there are exceptions. A wife's heavy drinking may be the factor which precipitates her husband's violence. It may also cause her to be the primary aggressor, and even precipitate her violence towards the children. Although men are more likely to be sexually aggressive when drunk, there is evidence that women can also be sexually provocative, demanding sexual relations when under the influence of alcohol.

Heavy drinking in women has been researched more sympathetically than has been the case with men. Premenstrual tension, gynaecological problems, the long-term effects of childhood sexual abuse or other forms of sexual attack, marital violence, and depressive features, either endogenous or reactive, are possible extenuating factors. In the context of marital violence it is easy to think of a cause for the female victim; but it must not be forgotten that there may also be problems in the marriage which cause men to drink heavily. They may, for example, feel trapped in the relationship and be unable to express their feelings and frustrations. Alcohol provides the release, and in some cases this removal of inhibitions is enough to allow the aggressive feelings to be translated into violence.

SUPPORT GROUPS

Although the first support group for battered wives was set up in the United Kingdom by Erin Pizzey in 1971, there is no doubt that in the United States more professional support has been developed. In the United Kingdom most of the support has come from voluntary organizations, and as a result facilities tend to be rather patchy. Some areas have well-developed shelters, or refuges, for battered wives and their children, many of which also provide a counselling service for the women, while in other areas there may be next to no facilities. The UK Select Committee on Violence in Marriage of 1975 made the recommendation that there should be one refuge place per 10 000 head of population, but it is clear that in many areas this target has not been met. Organization of the refuges is only loosely guided by the National Women's Aid Federation. Most local refuges pursue their own course and run as best they can on local support; but the National Federation at least provides some telephone support, in that it channels enquirers in the direction of local help.

In some areas professional organizations are becoming involved; but again, this depends on the energy and devotion to the cause of individual workers. Ideally in every area there should be a designated key worker who can be contacted when a crisis arises. This person's identity should be known to all health workers, and the mode of referral should be clear. Understandably the refuges are in most cases reluctant to make their location and telephone number too public for fear of abuse, and even attack, from a drunken and violent man. Like it or not, the police have found themselves in the front line when domestic violence occurs. In the past they have been repeatedly criticized for being unhelpful, but there is little doubt that they are often faced with a difficult and delicate task. Nevertheless great advances have been made, specific officers have been designated and trained, hopefully backed by their colleagues, and the establishment of local victim-support groups has done a great deal, not only to help the victim, but to bring about an increased awareness of the problem and a corresponding change in attitudes.

PRACTICAL MANAGEMENT

Once a diagnosis of marital violence has been made a decision has to be taken as to what emergency action is needed. The sympathetic Casualty Officer who decides to keep the patient in hospital overnight, even if the injuries under other circumstances would not warrant such a course, may make the establishment of a chain of intervention more possible. However, even this small step may be difficult, as the woman herself may be reluctant to accept admission, knowing she has left behind distressed children, perhaps with no suitable person to look after them. In most cases her husband, if he has dared to accompany her to hospital, will be reluctant to leave her alone in the presence of doctors and nurses, and will use every excuse to take her home. The cases which do reach hospital are in fact only the tip of the iceberg; many injuries will not receive the emergency attention they deserve, and others may not be sufficiently severe for hospitalization, but none the less represent a serious, and probably a recurring, problem.

The first decision which has to be made concerns the need to separate the two parties as a matter of urgency. If the police have made an immediate arrest, which is still quite rare, the violent man will only be kept in custody for a few hours, and in most cases will be returning to the marital home. It is possible that he will be served with a non-molestation order; but for this to be made into an exclusion order evidence is needed of further violence, or of the probablity of further violence. Even though there may have been a number of violent episodes in the past, and the injured woman is frightened of her situation, this does not easily translate into evidence which will stand up in court. Thus in many such situations the only emergency action available is for the woman and her children to seek the sanctuary of a refuge for battered wives (or Women's Aid Refuge, as they prefer to be called). This is a serious decision for any woman to make; perhaps she has contemplated leaving home on a number of occasions and has been deterred by the practical considerations of where to go with her children, but to voluntarily give up her home and to move herself and her children to a group home, with all its attendant lack of privacy and possible overcrowding, is not an easy step to take. Nevertheless, it offers the safety and support which many distressed women need at this particular time.

Clearly there are many women who can turn to their families for support at this time of crisis, and it is only when this is not possible that the Refuge becomes the only option. Not all families are in a position to be supportive: there may still be younger siblings, and literally no space for the battered wife and her children. Childless women obviously do not present such a problem, but even so the family may have its own difficulties in terms of broken relationships, and perhaps its own history of violence. There may be a lack of sympathy for the daughter in distress, particularly if she had been repeatedly warned against the relationship she entered into. It may even be that she embarked upon it in order to escape from unhealthy relationships at home, perhaps even incest.

All these major decisions have to be taken by what may well be a very emotionally disturbed woman. It is quite probable that she may be suffering from a post-traumatic stress disorder; but in any event, she is likely to experience considerable emotional problems for some time to come, even if she is adequately sheltered and supported and there is no repetition of violence.

Women who go to a Refuge

Some of the factors which make removal to a Refuge the best course of action for a battered wife have already been outlined. A Refuge, however, is not equipped for long-term residence; it is a crisis centre, which aims to help the woman to sort out her legal, financial, and accommodation problems, although in reality it does far more than this by providing the group support of other women in the same predicament. Unfortunately the hoped-for short-term residence often becomes longer than is either expected or desired: legal problems, for example, can take time to resolve; but undoubtedly it is the matter of alternative accommodation which presents the greatest long-term problem. Obviously if the parties are to be separated they both need homes; but the question of who is to pay for the second home inevitably arises, and in these circumstances the husband is usually reluctant to do so, or may of course be unable to do so. The problem is thus presented to hard-pressed Housing Departments, with their long waiting-lists and limited resources, and as time goes by there is an increase in the avoidable pressures upon the woman to return to the marital home. But many women who do return home are subjected to further violence, and in one-third of cases these attacks are rated as life-threatening.

Women who return to the marital home

In some ways the woman who returns to live with the man who was violent towards her needs even more support than does the woman who separates from her violent partner. Unfortunately this is not likely to be forthcoming, as it is usually assumed that once the crisis has settled there will be a reconciliation and a return to normality. This, however, is usually simply wishful thinking, with no basis in reality, and is really no more than a convenient excuse for inactivity.

The fact that violence has become known to professionals may in some circumstances lessen the likelihood of its further repetition; but nothing has really changed, and most of the information available indicates that the violence will usually begin again.

Where the problem of violence is clear it would be negligent not to attempt treatment. Alcoholism in the man is the most common precipitant of violence; but without the alcoholic acknowledging this there is no hope of change. Morbid jealousy has been recognized as a dangerous pathology for which there may be a variety of causes. Where these are clear they should be treated; but experience has shown that in the majority of cases the morbid jealousy is part of the overall personality. Husbands often submit to treatment in an attempt to bring about a reconciliation; but regretfully the treatment they choose may not be appropriate – for example, hypnosis for personality disorder. In the United States treatment programmes for both men and women have been recommended. Group support is seen as being more effective than individual counselling alone, but even so there are many problems that cannot be dealt with in groups: every battered wife, for example, needs the support of a specific adviser who will monitor the overall situation. Women who attend a victim-support group learn not to simply accept their situation: thus, their first task is to unlearn learned helplessness. Most groups use some form of assertiveness training; but where there has been marital violence this can precipitate further violence.

Ideally, if the woman is to attend a group, then so should the man; but this is even more difficult to organize, and as a consequence few groups of this type exist. Treatment aims should be the teaching of communication skills and of self-control, and it has been suggested that after the initial treatment in separate groups the couple should move on to a mixed group of both men and women. All this, however, needs careful organization and control.

Marital therapy still remains a favourite form of treatment, provided that the couple agree to attend and a therapist can be found who will be sympathetic to the problem. Here the dynamics of the relationship can be explored, and perhaps changes can be made on either side which are acceptable to both parties and can lead to control of the anger and the prevention of further violence.

Primary prevention

One might hope that much has been achieved as a result of the increasing public awareness of marital violence. It does seem that attitudes are changing: certainly it is no longer seen as a man's right to hit his wife if he so wishes. At one time he might have received some measure of support from his peers for his actions, but this no longer seems to be the case; and, where marital violence was once accepted as the norm in some families, increasing publicity has made it clear that this is not a pattern of behaviour which has to be tolerated. Women are collectively asserting themselves and are using the avenues of escape which have now been made known, while the men who want to continue this way of life are becoming more isolated and can expect to have to live without a female partner. In combating the continued cycle of violence, which is passed from generation to generation in some families, this educational approach seems to be the most powerful weapon.

Relationship to other family violence

With the development of studies in child abuse, marital violence, and the more recent study of the abuse of elderly relatives, it is becoming increasingly clear that all have features in common. Violence appears to breed violence, and being the victim of violence as a child leads to violence in the next generation, with the victim becoming the aggressor. This aggression may be directed at a wife or at children, and we are now seeing that it can go full circle, and can include the elderly members of a family. For some women their life may be that of a perpetual victim, first as a child and then as a wife. Women who are the victims of marital violence may take their frustration out on their children, and men who are violent to their wives may extend their aggression to their children.

The temper tantrums which can be observed amongst some of the children at a refuge for battered wives are truly alarming, and in the older children it is easy to see how some of these aggressive young males will become the wife-batterers of the future.

The way in which the violence is transmitted from one generation to the next is understood to some extent (see Chapter 9). Clearly there are both genetic factors and learned patterns of behaviour, although other factors play a part. There may be a defect in the social skills needed to deal with a crisis or a conflict situation. It is very common to draw on past family experience, and where violence has been used as a problem-solver in the past, then violence is likely to be used again. Thus in this sense it is a learned maladaptive pattern of behaviour. This is, of course, the hallmark of a personality disorder – a disorder which itself seems to be passed on in much the same way.

Because it has a common link, mention must again be made of alcoholism. Heavy drinking in men has been noted in the fathers of abused children, in men who batter their wives, and in men who abuse an elderly relative. Again, alcohol does not only affect men, and women who drink heavily may also abuse their children. Heavy drinking in the elderly, too, can release aggression in those who are forced to look after them and who have a history of responding to problems with violence.

SUMMARY

It is only in the past twenty years that we have at last begun to take the problem of family violence seriously, and, with the erosion of the secrecy with which it has traditionally been surrounded, the true extent of the problem is gradually becoming clear.

In some families, the seeds of violence, sown in childhood, are passed from generation to generation. Many women, subjected to violence in courtship, will end the relationship; but sadly, many more will continue, in the hope that things will improve, only to find, when they have children and escape is more difficult, that they have become battered wives.

Social, psychological, and personality factors in both parties allow this to occur; but in only a minority of cases is there treatable pathology.

Slowly we are learning some strategies which may help; but this is only possible where both parties are willing to co-operate, and where there appears to be a minimal danger of immediate repeated violence. Regretfully, in many cases the pathology is too serious, the relationship too damaged, and the danger of further violence too immediate to allow the couple to stay together. Where this is the case the only sane intervention is to separate the parties concerned, despite the problems this will lead to in rehabilitation.

There is no doubt that Hostels for Battered Wives have played a leading role in this field, and they may well continue to do so for some time to come, for it is only when society has learned that this is not an acceptable pattern of behaviour – and that message has got through to potentially violent men – that these Refuges will start to empty.

FURTHER READING

Binney, V., Harkell, J., and Nixon, J. (1981). *Leaving violent men*. National Women's Aid Federation, London.

Browne, K.D. (1989). Family violence: spouse and elder abuse. In *Clinical approaches to violence* (ed. K. Howells and C.R. Hollin). Wiley, Chichester.

Cobbe, F.P. (1878). Wife torture in England. *Contemporary Review*, **32**, 57–87.

Frieze, I.H. (1983). Investigating the causes and consequences of marital rape. *Journal of Women in Culture and Society*, **8**, 532–53.

McClintock, F.H. (1978). Criminological aspects of family violence. In *Violence and the family* (ed. J.P. Martin), Wiley, Chichester.

Mullen, P.E., Roman-Clarson, S.E., Walton, V.A., and Herbison, G.P. (1988). Impact of sexual and physical abuse on women's mental health. *Lancet*, **i**, 841–5.

Rosenburg, M.S. and Rossman, B.B.R. (1991). The child witness to marital violence. In *Treatment of family violence*. (ed. R.T. Ammerman and M. Hersen), Wiley, New York.

Shepherd M. (1961). Morbid jealousy. *Journal of Mental Science*, **107**, 687–753.

Stark, E. and Flitcraft, A. (1988). Violence among intimates: an epidemiological review. In *Handbook of family violence* (ed. V.B. Van Hasselt, A.S. Morrison, and M. Hersen), Plenum Press, New York.

8 Non-accidental injury of children

Alan Emond

HISTORICAL AND CULTURAL BACKGROUND

Children have been victims of violence since ancient times, and in all societies. Violence has been perpetrated against them in every conceivable manner: physically, emotionally, by sexual exploitation, through neglect, and by enforced labour. Exposure and infanticide have been near universal forms of child abuse over the years, allowing many societies to ensure that only healthy newborns survive. This freedom for parents to kill defective or unwanted babies continued in some parts of Europe until the nineteenth century. In 1885 the Society for the Prevention of Cruelty to Children reported the ways in which London children were battered: by boots, crockery, pans, shovels, straps, ropes, thongs, pokers, fire, and boiling water. Severe physical chastisement was regarded in Britain as an acceptable form of disciplining children until well after the Second World War. The introduction of the term 'battered child' in 1962 was thus a new name for a very old problem, but marked the beginning of increasing awareness and concern about violence towards children.

The most fundamental change that has taken place in society's attitude towards children in the last 40 years has been the acceptance (and now enshrinement in UK law under the Children Act 1989) that children are not the possessions of their parents, but have rights of their own.

In addition, it is now accepted that children require special protection because of their dependency on adults for care, and parents and society have a responsibility to meet their needs. However, violence towards children remains an enormous problem in Britain in the 1990s, and takes many forms. Non-accidental injury is merely the physical and most obvious manifestation of violence; but sexual abuse, emotional abuse, and neglect have equally damaging effects on children in the long term.

Although it is probable that violence towards children occurs in all societies, cross-cultural variability in child-rearing beliefs and practice make it difficult to define a universal standard for good child-care, abuse, and neglect. While cultures differ in their definitions of child-maltreatment, all societies have criteria for what constitutes acceptable behaviour towards children. In a society, like Britain, which is changing and becoming more multicultural, the boundaries of acceptable behaviour towards children in areas like discipline are also changing. Professionals who work with children require both a sensitivity to different rearing practices in families from different cultural and religious backgrounds, and also a clear understanding of the consensus of what is acceptable adult behaviour towards children.

Non-accidental injury in the family

The vast majority of non-accidental injuries take place in families. The family is paradoxically both the most physically violent group or institution that a typical citizen will encounter and also a group which children look to for love, support, and gentleness. Violence towards children cannot be separated from violence in families on a wider scale. The care-takers who abuse and injure children are most often biological parents, but may be step-parents, adoptive or foster parents, grandparents, siblings, or other relatives. Violence towards children is often linked to other violent behaviour in families, and is particularly associated with wife-battering. A recent study in Bristol UK, compared an Accident and Emergency Department Register of adult victims of violence with the Child Protection Register of children who had been physically abused. Women who had been the victims of domestic violence were shown to be significantly more likely to have their children registered for physical abuse. This research emphasized the importance of ensuring protection of the children of women who seek treatment for injuries sustained in assault.

The origins of violence in the family, and of its manifestations as non-accidental injury to children, are complex. For example, it is common for abusive parents to give a history of experiencing neglect or violence in their own childhood.

Inconsistent, unsympathetic care in childhood, with unrealistic demands, excessive criticism, and punishment for failure results in adults with poor self-esteem, poor basic trust, and a poor understanding of how to provide for a child's needs. Violent behaviour will manifest in such adults at times of stress, and if directed at children in the family will lead to patterns' being transmitted from parent to child – and so the potential for physical abuse, neglect, and sexual exploitation is transferred to another generation (see Chapter 9).

Physical injury to children is usually perpetrated by a care-taker who has a tendency to be violent which is related to his or her early life, and this is often directed at a child who is perceived in some way to be unsatisfactory. The child may be unwanted, or the wrong sex, or have the wrong facial features. The precipitant to the violence is often in a crisis of some sort, placing extra stress on a care-taker who is poorly supported and externalizes inner conflict and frustration as violent behaviour. The stress and conflict which characterizes certain families is a major factor in the non-accidental injury of children. However, violence is only one response to stress. The male predominance in perpetrators of violence to children reflects not just man's physical strength, but also his typical behavioural response to stress – while women tend to respond to stress by depression rather than violence.

Fathers who are physically violent to their children are more likely to have observed their own fathers hit their mothers. Higher rates of child abuse are found in families where adults believe that physical punishment and slapping a spouse are acceptable behaviour.

Certain groups of infants and children are at risk of being physically abused and neglected. Included in this group are normal infants who are the product of a difficult pregnancy or delivery, or are born from an unplanned pregnancy, of the wrong sex, of an unloved father, or during a period of severe family stress and crisis.

Infants who are perceived as 'abnormal' are particularly at risk, and these include infants who are significantly pre-term, those with congenital abnormalities, and those who have chronic illnesses or physical disability. A further group of children who can be particularly at risk of non-accidental injury are those who are described as 'difficult'. These children tend to be hyperactive, fussy and difficult to feed, have abnormal sleep patterns, cry excessively, and are perceived by their parents to be unresponsive to loving care.

However, although it is true that some children are extremely difficult and push their care-takers beyond their ability to cope, it is important not to stress the provocative behaviour of the child at the expense of disregarding the parent's own difficulties and deficiencies in care-taking.

PRESENTATION OF NON-ACCIDENTAL INJURIES IN CHILDREN

Fractures

The original description of the battered baby syndrome by Kempe in 1962 recognized the importance of any discrepancy between the parent's history and the child's clinical injuries, and highlighted the significance of multiple injuries in different sites and of different ages. Fractures to infants and young children should be treated with particular suspicion. Most accidental fractures in infants and toddlers result from falls from more than three feet, and are single, linear, or green-stick fractures of the child's long bones, or narrow parietal skull fractures. One study from Nottingham showed that all abused children with fractures were under five years of age, and 80 per cent were under 18 months. In contrast, 85 per cent of accidental fractures in children occurred after the age of five years. Abused children are much more likely to have associated soft-tissue bruising of the head and neck, or to have multiple injuries.

Other indicators of child abuse, such as failure to thrive or facial bruising, may be important cues in distinguishing non-accidental from accidental fractures.

Fractures following physical abuse occur in almost any bone, and child abuse cannot be diagnosed on the pattern of fractures alone. A careful history, including risk factors for abuse in the family, followed by a full examination, is essential for a correct diagnosis. When the injury, or the history, suggests physical abuse, or if the child is less than 18 months old, a skeletal survey will be necessary. This should be a complete radiographic survey of the child's skeleton, and should be reported by an experienced radiologist, as many cases of abuse have been diagnosed from fractures which are not clinically obvious. Such fractures may be old or healing, or the sites may be hidden (for example, in the ribs, pelvis, or skull).

Metaphyseal and epiphyseal fractures are the classic injuries of child abuse, caused by pulling and twisting forces from shaking the child by the arms and legs. Fragments of bone become separated from the ends of long bones, usually as a chip or as a whole plate. Although they only account for 10 per cent of fractures resulting from abuse, they are virtually diagnostic, as they are such uncommon accidental fractures.

Rib fractures strongly suggest physical abuse unless there is a clear history of trauma (for example crush injury). Deliberate rib fractures are caused by chest compression, which often occurs during the shaking of babies, or through punches or kicks delivered to older children. Rib fractures are often multiple, and occur posteriorly. Careful and expert radiological examination is required to detect some rib fractures. Recent fractures are especially difficult to identify, particularly at the costo-vertebral junction, and an isotope bone scan may be necessary to confirm them.

Accidental fractures of the shaft of long bones usually result from direct trauma, which causes a transverse break. Non-accidental fractures, however, often arise from indirect trauma – for example, being swung by the legs leads to spiral fractures. However, there is no clear distinction between long bone fractures arising from accidents and those arising from abuse. Other factors in the history, or the presence of other injuries, must be taken into account when considering the cause of long-bone fractures.

The discovery of multiple long-bone fractures, fractures of different ages, or injuries which are not reported by the carers, should raise suspicion of abuse. Thickening or elevation of the periosteum may be a pointer to a previously unrecognized fracture.

Sub-periosteal haemorrhage lifts the periosteum from the shaft of the bone, and this process often takes 10–14 days to appear radiographically. An experienced radiologist may be able to date fractures, as healing takes place through recognized stages of periosteal new-bone formation, soft callus, hard callus, and remodelling. A radiologist will also be helpful in confirming that the rest of the skeleton is radiologically normal, excluding uncommon but important genetic, metabolic, or bone diseases (for example, osteogenesis imperfecta).

In all cases of fracture where abuse is suspected, good communication is essential between the various professionals involved – casualty staff, radiologists, orthopaedic surgeons, paediatricians, and social workers – so that mistakes are not made in diagnosis. It is very important to avoid conflicting messages being given to the family, and to ensure that clear evidence is given to the Police and to the Courts. The child will need follow-up, not just to ensure that the fracture has healed satisfactorily, but also to consider his or her growth, development, and emotional needs.

Head injuries

Young children frequently sustain minor injuries, often to the forehead, when learning to walk or from bumping into furniture. Most of the injures to children under five who fall out of bed, prams, and couches do not result in skull fractures. Although fractures of the skull can occur after fairly minor falls, most accidental fractures have been shown to result from moderate falls of between 3 and 6 feet – for example, falling from a standing adults' arms. Skull fractures resulting from such accidents are usually linear and narrow, and characteristically affect the parietal bone. They are rarely associated with other intracranial injury (for example subdural haematoma). The parent may only realize that significant damage has been sustained when a hard swelling appears on the child's scalp one or two days later, and sometimes may have forgotten the original injury. Such late presentation may be viewed with suspicion, and requires careful evaluation by experienced paediatricians and radiologists to avoid a mistaken diagnosis of non-accidental injury.

Although parents who have abused their children often give a history of a minor fall or accident, the force actually used in physical abuse (violent shaking or hitting the child's head against a wall) is so much greater than that in common accidents that the pattern of injury is different. After abuse, skull fractures tend to be complex or multiple, involve more than one cranial bone, and cross more than one suture line.

Fractures of the temporal and frontal bones, and the thick bones at the base of the skull, are also much more likely to be due to violent abuse rather than an accident.

A useful indicator of abuse in young children is a measurement of the maximum width of the fracture. If the fracture is more than 5 mm wide, it is very likely to have been the result of child abuse, whereas accidental fractures are usually less than 1 mm in width. Growing or expanding skull fractures occur in infancy, and are associated with a dural tear and brain injury beneath the fracture. Such fractures are the result of a more serious blow to the head, and are much more likely to be associated with abuse. Subsequent enlargement of the fracture may form a cranial defect which requires surgical repair. The presence of a growing fracture, when the explanation given is a minor fall, should therefore raise suspicion of abuse.

Depressed fractures are very uncommon in young children, and indicate abuse unless a history is given of a fall on to a sharp object. A particularly characteristic injury is a depressed fracture of the frontal bone caused by hitting the child's head against the wall, the floor, or furniture.

Children who develop irritability, vomiting, or impaired consciousness after a seemingly trivial injury are likely to have been violently abused, and should be investigated by CT scanning. This may demonstrate a subdural haematoma, cerebral contusion, or cerebral oedema resulting from violent shaking. The presence of any of these signs is a reflection of the severity of the head injury, and is indicative of abuse. Subdural haematomas may occasionally arise after birth trauma, but usually present within the first few days of life, and do not result in chronic signs or symptoms. Subdural haematomas presenting outside the perinatal period indicate severe head injury, and in the absence of an adequate history are diagnostic of abuse.

However, children may suffer serious head injuries from abuse without there being any history of trauma or external signs of physical injury. Children who have sustained intracranial injury may present with unexplained neurological deficit, irritability, seizures, apnoeic attacks, or non-specific symptoms, such as feeding problems. A careful history, neurological examination, skull

X-ray, lumbar puncture, and a CT scan may be helpful in the diagnosis.

Infants with head injuries, or those suspected to have been abused, should have a retinal examination after the pupils have been dilated. The presence of retinal haemorrhages without adequate explanation is strongly indicative of abuse, and is usually the result of shaking. Violent shaking causes cerebral oedema, and the underlying increase in intracranial pressure leads to increased pressure in the central retinal vein – resulting in multiple retinal haemorrhages.

Cerebral contusion, haemorrhage, and oedema lead to many of the deaths and much of the long-term disability resulting from physical abuse. Haemorrhage within the brain can directly damage cortical pathways (for example those concerned with vision), lead to infarction and cerebral atrophy, or result in post-traumatic hydrocephalus. It is thus particularly important to identify and protect children who are subject to violent abuse to the head.

Burns and scalds

Accidental burns and scalds of young children are unfortunately far too common, and reflect inadequate supervision or lack of awareness of the dangers that common domestic appliances pose to children. It is often difficult to distinguish between careless or ignorant parenting (which is a temporary lapse in the usual protection afforded to a child) and deliberate neglect (which is a deliberate failure to protect the child).

Deliberate burning or scalding of children can cause very significant injuries, and is usually used as a punishment or to provoke fear in the child. Such injuries may also be sadistic, and inflicted by an adult for excitement or sexual arousal. The separation of deliberate from accidental heat injuries is best made on the history and the behaviour of the parents. Parents whose children have accidentally burnt themselves will be anxious and guilty, and will want urgent treatment for their child. Abusive parents may lack concern, delay presentation of the injury, or tell a vague or changing story, or may be hostile and angry towards staff and refuse admission for treatment. Mothers who burn their children deliberately may themselves be depressed or seeking help, or have been themselves the victims of abuse. Children who have been deliberately injured may be withdrawn and passive, or excessively angry and rebellious.

Accidental burns and scalds are most common during the second year of life, when toddlers become more mobile, whereas the peak age for children being deliberately burnt is during the third year.

The reported incidence of deliberate heat injury is low (1–2 per cent of children admitted to hospital), but this form of violent abuse is almost certainly under-diagnosed and under-reported.

A hospital-based study in Leeds that compared accidental with deliberately-inflicted burns and scalds found that all the abused children were under 6 years of age, and that nearly half had additional injuries or were failing to thrive. Deliberate injuries typically affected the backs of the hands, the buttocks, the feet, and the legs. The injuries were incompatible with the history given. Scalds accounted for the majority of accidents, usually following spillage from kettles or saucepans. In these accidents the hot liquid usually scalds the front of the child's body, affecting the face, trunk, shoulders, or upper arms. In contrast, the most common way of deliberately scalding children is forced immersion in a bath or a sink. This form of violent injury typically affects the soles of the feet and the lower legs or the hands and arms in a stocking or glove distribution, without splash-marks. A clear tide-mark confirms that such scalds have been caused by forced immersion.

Dry contact burns from household appliances are common after both accidents and abuse. The usual site for accidental burns is the palm and tips of the fingers. Contact burns in unusual sites, showing the clear outline of an object, should give rise to suspicion of abuse. Deliberate cigarette burns are usually inflicted as punishment on the back of the hands, the arms, or the legs. Accidental brushing against a lighted cigarette causes a very superficial eccentrically-shaped burn, and not the well-defined circular mark of a deliberate cigarette burn.

An improvement in the recognition of deliberate injury by burning or scalding requires increased awareness by all who deal with children, and good liaison between hospital, primary-care team, social workers, and police. Visits to the home will be necessary to assess the circumstances of the injury, and to support the parents.

The characteristics of the children and their interaction with their parents may give useful insight into the dynamics which lead to violent abuse. Gaining the child's confidence may lead to a disclosure of what really happened.

Bruising

Careful examination of the bodies of most children who have learned to walk is likely to reveal some small bruises of different ages. These are typically found on the bony extensor surfaces, such as the shins, knees, and elbows, and the forehead. In exploring the world, and in normal play, healthy children frequently suffer minor injuries, and these usually heal without any sequelae or disability.

Children who have been physically abused often have minor soft-tissue bruises that have been dismissed or not noticed, and these may be the early warning of much more serious injuries. The most important rule when assessing bruises and scratches, and other injuries of the skin, is not to confuse the severity of the injury with its significance in terms of child abuse. For example, small round bruises on a baby's cheek may be trivial injuries which will quickly heal, but they could be highly significant if they are finger-marks from violent gripping and shaking. Some forms of bruising are characteristic of physical abuse – for example finger-marks, slap-marks, and bilateral black eyes. In most cases a careful evaluation is needed of the history, the parents' attitude, and the whole child – in terms of growth, development, and behaviour, as well as of the actual injury. Checking the Child Protection Register every time a child is seen with an injury may be a time-consuming process, but will help to identify children with repeated injury, and prevent the escalation of violent abuse leading to serious injury.

The site of injury may also be critical in determining whether or not a bruise is accidental. Bruises to the head and neck are particularly significant, and would support a non-accidental diagnosis if they affect soft tissues like the cheeks or the eyelids, or if they are multiple and of different ages.

Grip-marks are commonly seen at the angle of the jaw or on the cheek. Slap-marks are found on the face or the ears, often including fine haemorrhages. Black eyes may be acquired accidentally during playtime fights or by bumping into furniture, in which case the child can usually give an account of what happened. Bruising inside the bony rim of the orbit, bruising of different ages, or eye bruising for which no explanation can be given should arouse suspicion that the injury may be the result of adult violence.

In babies and toddlers injuries inside the mouth (a torn frenulum or bruising to the gums) may result from forced feeding, with a bottle or a spoon being rammed into the mouth – though again, such injuries alone are not diagnostic. In older children dislodged or broken teeth may be the result of accidental falls, but can also be caused by punches to the mouth, or by being pushed down the stairs. A high index of suspicion is required to identify cases of non-accidental injury in Casualty Departments and Dental Surgeries.

Violent sexual abuse

Sexual abuse is part of the spectrum of violence towards children. In one large group of children proven to have been sexually abused 15 per cent initially presented with bruising or other injury. Doctors who examine children as part of the assessment of non-accidental injury need to be aware of the overlap between physical and sexual abuse. However, most sexual abuse in childhood does not result in physical injury, or in abnormal physical signs on genital examination.

Bruising of the buttocks, the genital area, and the breasts may be associated with sexual abuse. Grip marks on the thighs, and symmetrical bruises around the knees, suggest sexual abuse with forceful gripping by the abuser. Bite marks or burns of breasts, abdomen, buttocks, or genitalia are often associated with sexual abuse. Laceration or scars in the hymen or loss of hymenal tissue are virtually diagnostic of forceful penetration. An enlarged hymenal opening, labial bruising or oedema, or vaginal discharge are supportive signs of, but are not diagnostic on their own, of violent sexual abuse.

Similarly, abnormalities of the anus should be interpreted with caution, and other supportive evidence is required to make a diagnosis of abuse. Fresh lacerations, with swelling, bruising, and congestion are strongly supportive of blunt penetrating trauma to the anus. Reflex anal dilatation, anal laxity, chronic anal fissures, and 'funnelling' of the anus are also seen in conditions not associated with abuse, and should be evaluated in conjunction with other evidence from a joint investigation with social services and the police.

Although injuries associated with sexual abuse may be horrific, the most long-term damage caused by such violence is emotional and psychological. Many studies from around the world have shown the long-term psychiatric and sexual morbidity suffered by women and men who have been sexually abused in childhood.

INTERVENTION AND TREATMENT

The identification of a non-accidental injury to a child is only the first stage in a process which needs to be founded on co-operation between different agencies. The first priority is to ensure that the child is protected in a 'place of safety', in hospital, in foster care, or in a safe family situation in the community. The period of separation of mother and child should be kept as short as possible whilst further investigations are carried out into the cause of the non-accidental injury and the underlying domestic situation. It may be necessary to apply to a family court for an Emergency Protection Order, which lasts for 8 days (and may be challenged in court after 72 hours).

Once the child's protection is assured, a case conference will need to be convened at the earliest opportunity, with an independant chairman not involved in the case. Representatives from social work, health, the police, and education will be invited, and have to provide written reports if they cannot attend. Good practice in multi-agency working in child abuse is described in *Working together* (DHSS 1988).

Good communication between the various agencies is essential, and should be combined with a respect for each other's differing roles in the assessment and management of the child and the family. The case conference is the forum to share concerns, in confidence, and to make a joint action plan which will be carried out by a 'core group' containing key workers from lead agencies involved with the family. The conference will also decide on whether to recommend that the child should be placed on the Child Protection Register (CPR), a decision which is usually ratified by an area-based review panel. It is now regarded as good practice to include one or both parents in the case conference discussions, and it is very important to ensure that only matters of substantiated fact are placed before the conference. The parents should also have the decisions of the conference confirmed in writing.

As part of the action plan, the case conference may wish to seek legal advice on the necessity of applying to the Court for a further legal order. Under the terms of the Children Act, the Court may only make such an order if it is concerned that the child is at risk of significant harm, and that the child's interests are better served by making an order than by not making one.

If the order involves further assessment of the child or of the parents, the Court is empowered to set a timetable for the assessment and a review date in court. The aims of the Children Act legislation are to encourage good multidisciplinary assessment with the minimum delay, to promote goal-directed treatment work with child and parents, and to keep 'out of home' placement as short as possible.

In the majority of cases of violent abuse, treatment of the child can begin as soon as the diagnosis is first suspected. Once the child's safety is secured, a treatment programme should be devised to replace what has been missing at home, and to modify behaviour patterns developed as a response to violent and unpredictable parenting. If the child is placed in temporary foster care, the foster parent will need advice, guidance, and support to deal with developmental delay and disturbed behaviour. If the abused child is kept in his or her own home, regular monitoring and support will be needed from social worker and health visitor. Pre-school children who have been abused often benefit from a structured day-nursery environment, which helps their development, behaviour, and relationships with peers, as well as with other adults.

The imposition of a consistent structure offers the child the opportunity to reduce anxiety, to develop impulse control, and to mature in behaviour. School-age children will need encouragement to talk about their experiences, and structured 'life history' counselling may help children come to terms with what has happened to them.

However, in order for the child's treatment to be effective, the parents must receive treatment as well. First, the abuser must acknowledge responsibility for the abuse and its impact on the child. Secondly, the extent to which family members have not adequately provided protection for each other is an important aspect of the acknowledgement process, and families may need help to move away from blaming one member for the violence. Thirdly, the individual who perpetrated the non-accidental injury will need help in recognizing his or her violent response to stress, and in establishing new patterns of parenting. All this takes time, appropriate help from committed and well-trained professionals, and the necessary resources (for example family centres). Unfortunately, adequate resources for treatment and rehabilitation of families in which violent abuse has occurred are lacking in most parts of the UK, and hard-pressed social service departments are forced to prioritize limited funds and manpower into child protection, rather than into treatment or rehabilitation.

The prevention of child abuse is an even more challenging task, which cannot be achieved by statutory provision alone. The Child Protection Registers (CPR) that are now held by every local authority in the UK are designed to facilitate the recognition of children who are at risk of abuse. The effectiveness of these registers depends on the awareness of all professionals who come into contact with children and effective communication between them. However, preventing child abuse within families requires changing parenting behaviour, and interrupting the trans-generational pattern of violent responses to stressful situations.

A comprehensive preventive service would include: all new parents receiving parenting education and support; all children receiving preventive education in schools; all parents under stress having access to self-help groups and other supportive services; and all victims of abuse having access to supportive help. Such preventive services are available only in skeleton form in many areas.

Although media coverage has resulted in increasing public concern about child abuse, more education and informed discussion is required to increase awareness of non-accidental injury of children, its causes, and its implications. Violent abuse of children will ultimately only be prevented if violent behaviour within families is reduced – and this requires fundamental changes in society.

FURTHER READING

Billmire, M.E. and Myers, S.A. (1985). Serious head injury in infants: accident or abuse? *Paediatrics*, **75**, 340–2.

Department of Health and Social Security and Welsh Office (1988). *Working together. A guide for inter-agency co-operation for the protection of children from abuse*. HMSO, London.

Helfer, R.E. and Kempe, R.S. (1987). *The battered child*, (4th edn). University of Chicago Press.

Hobbs, C.J. and Wynne, J.M. (1990). The sexually abused battered child. *Archives of the Diseases of Childhood*, **65**, 423–7.

Keen, J.H., Lendrum, J., and Wolman, B. (1975). Inflicted burns and scalds in children. *British Medical Journal*, **i**, 268–9.

Kempe C.H., Silverman, F.N. Steele, B.F. *et al.* (1962). The battered child syndrome. *Journal of the American Medical Association*, **181**, 17–24.

Meadow, R. (ed) (1989). *ABC of child abuse*. British Medical Journal, London.

Royal College of Physicians of London (1991). *Physical signs of sexual abuse in children*. The College, London.

Ward, L., Shepherd, J.P., and Emond, A.M. (1993). Relationship between adult victims of assault and children at risk of abuse. *British Medical Journal*, **306**, 1101–2.

Worlock, P., Stower, M., and Barbor, P. (1986). Patterns of fractures in accidental and non-accidental injury in children: a comparative study. *British Medical Journal*, **293**, 100–2.

9 The causes and prevention of offending, with special reference to violence

David P. Farrington

THE PREVALENCE AND NATURAL HISTORY OF OFFENDING

The aim of this chapter is to review knowledge about the causes and prevention of offending, with special reference to violence. 'Offending' in this chapter is defined to include the most common types of crimes that predominate in the official criminal statistics, namely theft, burglary, robbery, violence, vandalism, and drug use. Within a single chapter, it is impossible to review everything that is known about offending, and it is necessary to focus on the more important findings obtained in some of the better studies. Most research is concerned with offending by males. (For more detailed reviews of knowledge about offending, see Rutter and Giller, 1983; Wilson and Herrnstein, 1985. For more extensive knowledge about aggression and violence, see Pepler and Rubin, 1991.)

The Cambridge study

Special reference will be made to the Cambridge Study in Delinquent Development, which is a follow-up survey of 411 male Londoners from the age of 8 to the age of 32 (Farrington and West, 1990). At the time they were first contacted in 1961, the boys were all living in a working-class area of London. Most were then aged eight and on the registers of six state primary schools within a one-mile radius of a research office that had been established. Most were white in racial appearance and of British origin, since they were being brought up by parents who had themselves been reared in England, Scotland, or Wales. The boys were interviewed and tested in their schools when they were about 8, 10, and 14. They were interviewed in our research office at about 16, 18, and 21, and in their homes at about 25 and 32. On all occasions except at the ages of 21 and 25 the aim was to interview the whole sample;

and it was always possible to trace and interview a high proportion. For example, 95 per cent of those still alive were interviewed at 18, and 94 per cent at 32.

In addition to the interviews and tests with the boys, their parents were interviewed about once a year from when the boy was 8 until he was 14–15, in his last year of compulsory education. The boys' teachers also completed questionnaires when the boys were aged about 8, 10, 12, and 14. In addition, repeated searches were made in the Criminal Record Office to try to locate evidence of criminal convictions against the boys, their parents, their brothers and sisters, and (in recent years) their wives and cohabitants. However, official records were not the only sources of information about offending. Self-reports of offending from the boys themselves were obtained at every age from 14 onwards.

Prevalence of offending

The major violent offences are homicide (725 recorded by the police in England and Wales in 1991), (rape 4045), robbery (45 323), serious wounding or grievous bodily harm (9408), and other wounding or actual bodily harm (174 245; see Home Office, 1993). Violence, rape, and robbery accounted for just over 4 per cent of all offences recorded by the police in England and Wales in 1991 (about 230 000 out of 5 300 000). Less serious assaults ('common assaults') are non-indictable offences, and are not included in the figures for crimes or convictions. Roughly speaking, assault causing only bruises, scratches, swelling, or a black eye would be classified as common assault, while assault involving stabbing, shooting, broken bones, teeth knocked out, bleeding, or unconsciousness would be counted as wounding.

Legal definitions of offending can give rise to many problems. For example, the boundary between what is legal and what is illegal may be poorly defined and subjective, as when school bullying gradually escalates into criminal violence. Legal categories may be so wide that they include acts which are behaviourally quite different, as when robbery ranges from armed bank hold-ups carried out by gangs of masked men to thefts of small amounts of money perpetrated by one schoolchild on another. However, the advantage of legal definitions is that, because they are widely used, they permit the comparison of results obtained in different research projects.

The number of crimes recorded by the police in any year clearly under-represents the number of crimes actually committed. For example, in 1987, the major national victim survey (the 'British

Crime Survey') estimated that there were actually 566 000 woundings and 177 000 robberies, about five times the number of comparable offences recorded by the police (Mayhew *et al.*, 1989). In addition, the number of common assaults reported by victims was nearly 1 500 000. Taking wounding, robbery and common assault together, there were about six acts of violence with identifiable victims per 100 adults in England and Wales in 1987.

Criminal convictions are more prevalent than is usually realized. For example, a Home Office follow-up of a national sample of persons born in 1953 showed that 33 per cent of the males and 7 per cent of the females were convicted of 'standard list' offences (i.e. more serious or indictable offences, excluding motoring for example) up to the age of 30 (Home Office Statistical Bulletin, 1989*b*). Of the London males in the Cambridge Study, 37 per cent were convicted up to the age of 32, and 12 per cent were convicted of serious violent offences. However, again, the prevalence of convictions under-represents the prevalence of offending. According to their self-reports at different ages, 96 per cent of the London males had committed an offence at some time (burglary, theft, vandalism, assault, drug use, or fraud), and 70 per cent had committed an assault. Even at the age of 32, 37 per cent had struck someone in a fight in the previous five years, and 15 per cent of those living with a woman had hit their wife or cohabitant.

A typical violent incident

Many violent incidents consist of assaults between young males who have been drinking alcohol. Who is regarded as the 'offender' and who is regarded as the 'victim' may sometimes be a matter of chance. In the Cambridge Study, all our interviews were fully tape-recorded, making it possible to present verbatim reports of offences. Here is an illustrative account of a group fight by one boy at the age of 18 (from Farrington *et al.*, 1982a):

Got done for a fight up at the [pub]. I'd had only about – top whack – four pints, that's all. I was as sober as anything. I never usually drink round this area because they're all villains – everyone thinks they're Jack the Lad – you can tell the pubs – it was the [pub] – I used to go down there when I was young like and drink a lot in there but now I won't go into those sort of pubs – they're all young – the fellows I go around with are all older than me – they're all about 25 – so I wouldn't take them to any silly boys' pub – everyone wants to bash you on the nose if you look at them. You get these pubs about, don't you – silly boys – you can see them. It was about six months ago – I came out of the toilet – I was going to leave and go over the West End – I wasn't staying in there – and my mate – he drinks a lot in this [pub]. And as I came out of the toilet, this girl, she burnt me with a cigarette – she just caught me, like, and when you get burned it does hurt, doesn't it? Fuck me. I turned round and the bloody geezer she was with – a right Jack the Lad – I said 'You could at least say fucking sorry, can't you?' I did get a bit needled. He says 'Oh piss off,' like. So I started arguing. Then my mate, Johnny, he walks over – he says 'What's the matter?' I said 'Nothing, like. She burnt me and she didn't say sorry, like.' Johnny said to him 'Look pal, you step outside and we'll settle it outside.' And he says 'No, I don't want a fight.' Well, I said 'Fucking don't be so flash about it then.' Anyway, the next thing I know I was just going to walk away and this bloody geezer – massive-sized geezer – hit me right over the nose with a bottle – it's another guy – this guy's mate. I didn't know him – I didn't know he was standing there – he hit me right over the nose with a bottle – I didn't know what happened – the next thing everyone's at the off – I'm so popular – I know everyone in the pub – so I get a lot of helping out – the next thing I know, my mate Johnny who got nicked with me – 28 stitches up his arm – the geezer smashed a bottle trying to put it in his face – he stopped it with his arm. The two geezers – when they got outside like – we had a fight with them and we gave them a right hiding – and one's seriously ill – nearly died – and the other one got 18 stitches in his head and all this – cut to pieces like – it wasn't done by me. Me and my mate – we went up to the hospital then – he's got his arm, and all my face is done in – there was only two of them so we walked away from the pub really – and these fellows done them in outside the pub. We had a couple of fights with them, but we left it – we said 'Leave it at that'; but they was carrying on like. There was only three of them other fellows who got hurt. We walked away because Johnny was pouring with blood, and my face – I've got no scars but it just cut open there like [bridge of nose] – so much blood it was unbelievable. We got down the hospital – we was down there about an hour and the police come down – they took us all in – there was an identity parade – one of the boys picked us out. They nicked us – we didn't have a leg to stand on but we're fighting the case – we want to charge them with GBH [grievous bodily harm] and all. We got done for maliciously wounding – not GBH. They were cut by a bottle but neither of us did it. We're fighting it in court. We went to court the other day and we said that we want a judge and jury. We've got solicitors and we're going to fight them. It'll come up after Christmas, it will.

This account shows how violent incidents escalate from small beginnings, as 'macho' young males react to minor irritations by confrontation rather than conciliation. The police account of the incident was as follows:

On [date] at 12.35 am at [place], committed by attacking one [the victim], hitting about the head and back with a broken beer glass. After an argument in the [—] public house, a fight started between the accused and another youth, also charged, and [the victim]. The fight was stopped by people in the bar. [The victim] and his girlfriend left the bar to go home. As they walked down [place], they were attacked by the accused and his codefendant. [The victim] was knocked to the ground, kicked and cut with a bottle. Police arrived at the scene in time to see the two accused running away. They were later seen at [—] hospital and arrested.

This boy pleaded not guilty to unlawful wounding and was found guilty only of common assault. Consequently, we did not count this offence as a conviction. Interestingly, in later life he was charged on two separate occasions with serious robberies of jewellery and silverware, but was found not guilty both times. However, he did have convictions for assaulting the police, unlawfully possessing a police truncheon, and unlawfully possessing ammunition (as well as three burglary convictions).

Versatility and continuity in offending

While the acts included in crimes are varied, it nevertheless makes sense to understand the characteristics of offenders. This is because offenders do not usually specialize in particular kinds of offence. In other words, people who commit one type of offence have a tendency also to commit other types. For example, in the Cambridge Study, 43 out of 50 convicted violent offenders also had convictions for non-violent offences (up to the age of 32).

More importantly, violent offences (and indeed other types of offences) seemed to be committed almost at random in criminal careers. As the males committed more and more offences, sooner or later they would commit a violent offence. Violent offenders tended to be persistent or frequent offenders, and they were indistinguishable in the Cambridge Study from other persistent offenders who had not been convicted of violence: in childhood, adolescence, and adulthood. Consequently, the causes of violence (or rather, of the potential to commit violent offences) must be the same as the causes of frequent and persistent antisocial and criminal behaviour. Violent offenders are extreme offenders, and it is not necessary to propose a theory specifically to explain the development of a violent person, as opposed to the development of offenders in general.

In addition, there is considerable continuity in offending over time, for example, between the juvenile and adult years. In the Cambridge Study, nearly three-quarters of those convicted as juveniles (age

10–16) were reconvicted between the ages of 17 and 24, and nearly half the juvenile offenders were reconvicted between the ages of 25 and 32. The males first convicted at the earliest ages tended to become the most persistent offenders, in committing larger numbers of offences at high rates over long time-periods.

Offending and antisocial behaviour

Just as offenders are versatile in their types of offending, they are also versatile in their antisocial behaviour generally. In the Cambridge Study, it has been argued that offending (which is dominated by crimes of dishonesty) is only one element of a larger syndrome of antisocial behaviour which arises in childhood and usually persists into adulthood. Hence valid implications about offending can often be drawn from research on child antisocial behaviour or conduct disorder.

The typical male offender tends to be born in a low-income, large-size family and to have criminal parents. When he is young, his parents supervise him rather poorly, use harsh or erratic child-rearing techniques, and are likely to be in conflict and to separate. At school, he tends to have low intelligence and attainment, is troublesome, hyperactive, and impulsive, and tends to be a bully, a frequent liar, and a truant. He tends to associate with friends who are also delinquents. By the age of 18, offenders tend to be antisocial in a wide variety of respects, including heavy drinking, frequent fighting, heavy smoking, reckless driving, using prohibited drugs, and heavy gambling. They have low-status job-records punctuated by periods of unemployment. In addition, they tend to be sexually promiscuous, often beginning sexual intercourse under the age of 15, have had several sexual partners by the age of 18, and usually have unprotected intercourse (Farrington and West, 1990).

These results from the Cambridge study are entirely consistent with those obtained in numerous other studies (see Farrington, 1992). For example, in a St Louis survey of black males, offending tended to be associated with truancy, precocious sex, drinking, and drug use. In Philadelphia, troublesome behaviour in *Kindergarten* (at the age of 3–4) predicted later police contacts; and in Chicago teachers' ratings of aggressiveness in the first grade (age 6) predicted self-reported offending at the age of 15.

The Cambridge Study extends these conclusions up to the age of 32. By that time, offenders tend to be separated or divorced from their wives and separated from their children. They tend to be unemployed or in low-paid jobs, to move house frequently, and to live in rented rather than owner-occupied accommodation. Their lives are still characterized by more evenings out, more heavy drinking and drunk driving, more violence, and more drug-taking than their contemporaries. Hence, the typical offender tends to provide the same kind of deprived and disrupted family background for his own children that he experienced, thus perpetuating from one generation to the next a range of social problems of which offending is only one element.

Age and crime

The prevalence of offending increases to a peak in the teenage years and then decreases in the twenties. The peak age of official offending for English males was 15 until 1987, but it increased to 18 in 1988 as a result of a decrease in recorded juvenile shoplifting offenders. The peak age for females was 14 until 1985 but then increased to 15. In England and Wales in 1991, the rate of findings of guilt or cautions of males for indictable offences increased from six per 1000 at the age of 10 to 67 at the age of 15 and a peak of 84 at the age of 18, and then decreased to 65 at the age of 20 and 30 at the age of 25–29. The corresponding figures for females were one per 1000 at the age of 10, a peak of 22 at the age of 15, 15 at 18, 11 at 20, and six at 25–29 (Home Office, 1993).

In the Cambridge Study, the rate of convictions increased to a peak at the age of 17 and then declined. It was 17 per 1000 at the age of 10, 68 at 17, 101 at 22, and 42 at 30. The median age for the commission of most types of offences (burglary, robbery, theft of and from vehicles, shoplifting) was 17, while it was 20 for violence and 21 for fraud. While the cumulative prevalence of convictions was high (37 per cent up to age 32), it was nevertheless true that only 6 per cent of the sample – the 'chronic' offenders – accounted for nearly half the convictions.

Self-report studies also show that the most common types of offending decline from the teens to the twenties. In the Cambridge Study, the prevalence of burglary, shoplifting, theft of and from vehicles, theft from slot machines, and vandalism all decreased from the teens to the twenties, but the same decreases were not seen for theft from work, assault, drug abuse, and fraud. The prevalence of assault, for example, was only slightly less at the age of 27–32 than at 15–18.

Many theories have been proposed to explain why offending peaks in the teenage years (see Farrington, 1986). For example, offending has been linked to testosterone levels in males, which increase during adolescence and early adulthood and decrease thereafter (e.g. Gove,

1985), and to changes in physical abilities or opportunities for crime. The most popular explanation focuses on social influence. From birth, children are under the influence of their parents, who generally discourage offending. However, during their teenage years, juveniles gradually break away from the control of their parents and become influenced by their peers, who may encourage offending in many cases. After the age of 20, offending declines again as peer influence gives way to a new set of family influences hostile to offending, originating in spouses and cohabitants.

Gender and crime

In general, males commit offences more frequently and seriously than females. In England and Wales in 1991 the male: female ratio for findings of guilt or cautions for indictable offences was about 5:1 (Home Office, 1993). However, this ratio was higher for serious offences such as burglary (about 23:1) and violence (about 7:1).

Other surveys of official records yield similar results. In a national English longitudinal survey of over 5000 children born in one week of 1946 (Wadsworth, 1979), 13 per cent of males and 2 per cent of females were convicted or cautioned for indictable offences up to the age of 20, giving a gender ratio of about 6:1. As has already been mentioned, in the Home Office follow-up of a national sample of people born in 1953, 33 per cent of males and 7 per cent of females were convicted up to the age of 30, giving a gender ratio of about 5:1. Similarly, in a follow-up of 2300 Inner London children by Ouston (1984), 29 per cent of males and 6 per cent of females were convicted or cautioned for an offence up to the age of 17–18, again giving a gender ratio of about 5:1.

Self-reported offending surveys yield much lower male:female ratios. However, most of the acts included in these surveys were relatively trivial. The gender ratio was higher for more serious acts such as burglary (15:1) in the largest survey reported by Campbell (1981) and carrying a weapon intending to use it (about 3:1).

Numerous explanations of gender differences in offending have been proposed. For example, they may have a biological foundation. Gender differences in aggressiveness are found very early in life, before any differential reinforcement of aggression in boys and girls (Maccoby and Jacklin, 1974). Furthermore, males are more aggressive than females in all human societies for which evidence is available, similar gender differences in aggressiveness are found in non-human primates as in humans, and aggression is related to levels of sex hormones such as testosterone. It seems obvious that, because on average males are bigger and stronger than females,

males will be better able to commit offences that require physical strength.

Not all offences are linked to aggression or physical strength, of course. Another possible explanation is that boys and girls are brought up differently by their parents. Generally, girls are supervised more closely, and girls stay at home more. Hence, if they behave in a socially disapproved fashion, their parents are more likely to notice this and react to it. Adults are generally more tolerant of incipient delinquency in boys than in girls, and they may encourage boys to be tough and take risks. On the theory that the strength of the conscience depends on the reinforcement of appropriate behaviour and the punishment of socially disapproved acts, it follows that girls will develop a stronger conscience and will be less likely to commit delinquent acts than boys.

The gender ratio can also be explained by reference to sex roles, social habits, and opportunities. Boys are more likely than girls to spend time hanging around on the street at night, especially in groups, and therefore are more likely to commit acts such as burglary and violence, which may often arise in this social situation. Girls are more likely than boys to spend time shopping, and so it is not surprising that shoplifting is the most common female offence. Boys have more interest in cars and weapons and more knowledge about how to use them, and so are more likely to commit car thefts and robberies. Later on in life, women have more opportunity to commit minor frauds because they are more likely to be collecting welfare benefits, and men are more likely to have the opportunity to steal from employers.

Race and crime

Most research on ethnic origin has compared blacks (Afro-Carib-beans) and whites. Blacks are more likely to be arrested than whites, especially for violent offences and particularly for robbery. For example, the Home Office Statistical Bulletin (1989a) shows that, of those arrested for robbery in London in 1987, 41 per cent were white, 54 per cent were black, 2 per cent were Asian, and 3 per cent were other or not known. These figures can be compared with the estimated resident population of London aged 10 or over, which at that time was 85 per cent white, 5 per cent black, 5 per cent Asian, and 5 per cent other or not known. The comparison of these figures gives a black:white ratio for robbery of 22:1. This ratio is increasing over time, since it was only 11:1 in 1977. The comparable American ratio for arrests for robbery was 10:1 in 1988, and this has stayed tolerably constant since 1976. The American black: white ratio in 1988 for all arrests for crimes of violence was 5:1, and for all arrests for serious ('index') offences was 3:1.

It might be argued that police arrests reflect bias against blacks. However, the black:white ratio based on victim reports of the offender's appearance seems, if anything, even higher. For example, in 1985 (the last year for which this information was compiled), London robbery victims said that their offenders were white in 19 per cent of cases, non-white in 56 per cent, mixed in 7 per cent and not known in the remaining 18 per cent (again according to Home Office figures). Making the plausible assumption that very few of the non-whites were not black, the black:white ratio corresponding to these figures is about 50:1. The discrepancy between the 50:1 ratio from victims and the 22:1 ratio from arrests may mean that the average black robber commits twice as many robberies as the average white robber, or that white robbers are twice as likely to be arrested as black robbers.

Longitudinal surveys yield lower black:white ratios, at least for prevalence. This is because prevalence ratios are constrained by the maximum of 100 per cent, whereas ratios like those above, based on numbers of offences, have no such constraint. In the first Philadelphia follow-up of 10 000 males born in 1945, 50 per cent of black males and 29 per cent of white males had police records for non-traffic offences by the eighteenth birthday (Tracy *et al.*, 1985). The comparable figures for the second cohort (born in 1958) were 42 per cent and 23 per cent. Up to the age of 30, 69 per cent of black males and 38 per cent of white males in the first cohort had police records for non-traffic offences (Wolfgang *et al.* 1987). Clearly, if 38 per cent of whites are arrested, the maximum possible black:white ratio is 100/38 or 2.6:1. Extensive reviews of the prevalence of officially recognized offending (e.g. Visher and Roth, 1986) show consistent black – white differences in the United States averaging about 3:1 over the majority of offences.

The most reliable English survey figures on ethnicity and crime are probably those obtained in Janet Ouston's (1984) follow-up of Inner London children. She found that 39 per cent of black males were convicted or cautioned as juveniles, in comparison with 28 per cent of white males. There are no comparable figures for Asians (those originating in India, Pakistan, or Bangladesh). However, studies elsewhere in England suggest that they have a lower crime rate than whites. Mawby *et al.* (1979) found that the annual rate for convictions and cautions in Bradford per 100 juveniles was about 3.2 for Asians and 6.3 for others (mostly whites).

The weight of evidence indicates that Afro-Caribbeans are more likely to commit offences – especially violent crimes – than whites, both in England and in the United States. Most theories proposed to explain black – white differences suggest that ethnicity in itself is not an important causal factor, but that blacks and whites differ on known precursors of offending such as low family income, poor parental child-rearing behaviour, or low intelligence. In an Inner London survey (Rutter *et al.*, 1975b), the socio-economic deprivation suffered by black families has been described especially with regard to poorer-quality housing and lower-status jobs. Partly because of the high proportion of black single-parent female-headed households, parental control and supervision has been found to be poor in black families (Wilson and Herrnstein, 1985). It has been suggested that black – white differences in the prevalence of offending reflect black – white differences in intelligence (Gordon, 1987). In testing these and other theories, it is important to determine whether observed ethnic differences in offending hold independently of these known precursors. For example, black – white differences in official offending have not always been shown to be independent of differences in social class or school attainment (Ouston, 1984).

In general, research on the link between ethnicity and offending has paid too little attention to ethnic groups other than whites and blacks. Results obtained with Orientals in the United States and with Asians in England suggest that minorities (even those suffering socio-economic deprivation) can be less delinquent than the majority white population, and it is important to establish why this is so. The low offending rate of Japanese-Americans has often been attributed to their closely-knit family system, characterized by strong parental controls; and a similar explanation has been proposed for the low offending rate of Asians in England. Thus, different child-rearing techniques might explain differential offending rates by ethnic groups.

PREDICTORS AND CORRELATES OF OFFENDING

Biological factors

Studies of twins and adopted children suggest that there is some kind of genetic influence on offending (Eysenck and Gudjonsson, 1989). This is indicated by the greater concordance (similarity) of monozygotic (identical) than dizygotic (fraternal) twins in offending. It might be argued that identical twins behave more identically because they are treated more similarly in their social environment, not because of their greater genetic similarity. Against this, however, the research of Bouchard *et al.* (1990) showed that identical twins reared apart were as similar in many respects (for example intelligence, personality, attitudes) as identical twins reared together. Also, it has been found that the offending of adopted children is more similar to that of their biological parents than to that of their adoptive parents (Mednick *et al.*, 1983), again suggesting some kind of genetic influence.

Numerous psychophysiological and biochemical factors have also been linked to offending. It has been concluded that offenders have a low level of arousal according to their low alpha activity on the EEG, or according to autonomic nervous system indicators such as heart rate, blood-pressure, or skin conductance (Venables and Raine, 1987). For example, in Scandinavian research, Magnusson (1988) found that adult offenders had low adrenaline levels at the age of 13, and Olweus (1987) showed that aggressive juveniles tended to have low adrenaline levels. The causal links between low autonomic arousal, consequent sensation-seeking, and offending are brought out in the theory of 'transient criminality' by Mawson (1987).

Heart rate was measured in the Cambridge Study at the age of 18. A low heart rate correlated with convictions for violence, but was not related to offending in general. Other physical measures taken in this research showed that relatively small boys were significantly more likely to be convicted than others. In addition, being tattooed was highly related to offending in the Cambridge Study. While the meaning of this result is not entirely clear, tattooing may reflect risk-taking, daring, and excitement-seeking.

Numerous prenatal and perinatal factors also predict a child's antisocial behaviour, including pregnancy and birth complications, low birth weight, and teenage parenting. In Denmark, birth-delivery complications predicted later violent offending (but not later property offending), especially for those with antisocial or psychiatrically disturbed parents (Kandel and Mednick, 1991).

Personality and impulsivity

One of the best known theories linking personality and offending was proposed by Hans Eysenck (1977). He viewed offending as rational behaviour, and assumed that a person's criminal tendency varied inversely with the strength of the conscience, which was a conditioned anxiety response that was built up in a process of conditioning. Eysenck concluded that offenders tended to be those who had not built up strong consciences. He also predicted that those who were high on Extraversion (E), Neuroticism (N), and Psychoticism (P) would tend to have the weakest consciences, and hence were the most likely to be offenders.

Studies relating Eysenck's personality dimensions to offending have been reviewed (Farrington *et al.*, 1982*b*). It was concluded that high N (but not E) was related to official offending, while high E (but not N) was related to self-reported offending. High P was related to both, since many of the items on the P scale are connected with antisocial behaviour (for example 'Have you had more trouble than most?'). However, in the Cambridge Study, when individual items of the personality questionnaire were studied, it was clear that the significant relationships were caused by the items measuring impulsivity (for example 'Do you generally do and say things quickly without stopping to think?'). Hence it was concluded that the major contribution inspired by the Eysenck theory was to identify the link between impulsivity and offending.

This link is also shown by the fact that offenders, and boys convicted of violence, tend to be lacking in concentration, restless, and daring in school. Farrington *et al.* (1990) developed a combined measure of hyperactivity-impulsivity-attention deficit (HIA) at the age of 8–10, and showed that this significantly predicted juvenile convictions independently of conduct problems at the age of 8–10. Hence, it might be concluded that HIA is not merely another measure of antisocial tendency. Other studies have also demonstrated that hyperactivity and conduct disorder are different. Sensation-seeking is also related to offending, and low self-control is the central feature of a recent theory of crime (Gottfredson and Hirschi, 1990).

It has been has argued that early infant temperament is a risk factor for later violence. When confronted with unfamiliar situations, some two-year-old children tend to be shy and inhibited, whereas others tend to be fearless and uninhibited. These temperamental differences at the age of two tend to be stable at least up to the age of seven (Kagan *et al.*, 1988). Furthermore, uninhibited children have lower heart rates than inhibited children, and a fearless, uninhibited temperament tends to predict later aggressiveness. Conversely, fearfulness may act as a protective factor, so that children from criminogenic families and communities who are fearful and inhibited tend not to become antisocial and violent.

Intelligence

The predictors of male delinquency have been reviewed (Loeber and Dishion, 1983) and it has been concluded that poor parental child-management techniques, offending by parents and siblings, low intelligence and educational attainment, and separations from parents were all important predictors. Longitudinal and other surveys have consistently demonstrated that children with low intelligence are disproportionally likely to become offenders.

In the Cambridge Study, about one-third of the boys scoring 90 or less on a non-verbal intelligence test (Raven's Progressive Matrices) at the ages of 8–10 were convicted as juveniles – twice as many as among the remainder. Low non-verbal intelligence was highly correlated with low verbal intelligence (vocabulary, word comprehension, verbal reasoning) and with low school attainment, and all these measures predicted convictions in general and convictions for violence to much the same extent. In addition to their poor school performance, offenders tended to be frequent truants, to leave school at the earliest possible age (which was then 15), and to take no school examinations.

Low non-verbal intelligence was especially characteristic of those convicted more than once, and of those first convicted at the earliest ages (10–13). Furthermore, low intelligence and attainment predicted self-reported offending almost as well as convictions, suggesting that the link between low intelligence and delinquency was not caused by the less intelligent boys having a greater probability of being caught. Similar results have been obtained in other projects (Wilson and Herrnstein, 1985).

The key explanatory factor underlying the link between intelligence and offending is probably the ability to manipulate abstract concepts. People who are poor at this tend to do badly in intelligence tests such as the Matrices (see above) and in school attainment, and they also tend to commit offences, mainly because of their poor ability to foresee the consequences of their offending and to appreciate the feelings of victims (i.e. their low empathy). Certain family backgrounds are less conducive than others to the development of abstract reasoning. For example, lower-class, poorer parents tend to live for the present and to have little thought for the future, and tend to talk in terms of the concrete rather than the abstract. A lack of concern for future consequences is also linked to the concept of impulsivity.

Modern researchers are studying not just intelligence but also detailed patterns of thinking and neuropsychological deficits. For example, in a New Zealand study of over 1000 children from birth to the age of 15, Moffitt and Silva (1988) found that self-reported offending was related to verbal, memory, and visual-motor integration deficits, independently of low social class and family adversity. Neuropsychological research might lead to important advances in knowledge about the link between brain functioning and offending. For example, the 'executive functions' of the brain, located in the frontal lobes, include sustaining attention and concentration, abstract reasoning and concept formation, anticipation and planning, self-monitoring of behaviour, and inhibition of inappropriate or impulsive behaviour. Deficits in these executive functions are conducive to low measured intelligence and to offending.

Family influences

Review of family factors as correlates and predictors of juvenile conduct problems and delinquency (Loeber and Stouthamer-Loeber, 1986) shows that poor parental supervision or monitoring, erratic or harsh parental discipline, marital disharmony, parental rejection of the child, and low parental involvement with the child (as well as antisocial parents and large family-size) have all been important predictors. Recent research (Widom, 1989) has also demonstrated the link between being physically abused or neglected as a child and committing violent offences later in life. Interestingly, this effect holds for blacks rather than whites and for males rather than females, and physical neglect was just as good a predictor of later violence as physical abuse.

In the Cambridge Study, it was found that harsh or erratic parental discipline, cruel, passive, or neglecting parental attitude, poor supervision, and parental conflict, all measured at the age of eight, all predicted both convictions in general and convictions for violence in particular. Poor parental child-rearing behaviour (a combination of discipline, attitude, and conflict), poor parental supervision, and low parental interest in education all predicted not only convictions but also self-reported offending. Poor parental child-rearing behaviour was related to early rather than later offending, and was not characteristic of those first convicted as adults.

Other studies also show the link between family factors and delinquency. In a Birmingham survey, the most important correlate of convictions, cautions, and self-reported offending was lax parental supervision (Wilson, 1980). A national survey of juveniles aged 14–15 and their mothers (Riley and Shaw, 1985), found that poor parental supervision was the most important correlate of self-reported offending for girls, and that it was the second most important for boys (after delinquent friends).

'Broken homes', involving permanent separation from a parent, also predict offending. In the Cambridge Study, both permanent and temporary (more than one-month) separations from parents before the age of 10 predicted later convictions and self-reported offending, providing that they were not caused by death or hospitalization. However, homes broken before the age of six were not unusually criminogenic.

Criminal, antisocial, and alcoholic parents tend to have delinquent sons. In the Cambridge Study, the concentration of offending in a small number of families was remarkable: less than 5 per cent of the families were responsible for about half the criminal convictions of all family members (fathers, mothers, sons, and daughters). Having convicted mothers, fathers or brothers by a boy's tenth birthday significantly predicted his own later convictions, including convictions for violence. Furthermore, convicted parents and delinquent siblings predicted self-reported offending as well as convictions. Unlike most early precursors, convicted parents were related less to offending of early onset (10–13) than to later offending. Also, convicted parents predicted which juvenile offenders went on to become adult criminals and which offenders by the age of 19 persisted in offending in their twenties.

These results are consistent with the psychological theory that offending occurs when the normal social learning process, based on rewards and punishments from parents, is disrupted by erratic discipline, poor supervision, parental disharmony, and unsuitable (antisocial or criminal) parents. However, some part of the link between criminal parents and delinquent sons may reflect genetic influences.

Peer influences

Generally, offences tend to be committed by small groups (of two or three people, usually) rather than by people acting alone (Reiss and Farrington, 1991). In the Cambridge Study, most officially recorded juvenile and young adult offences were committed with others, but the incidence of co-offending declined steadily with age from 10 onwards. Burglary, robbery, and theft from vehicles were particularly likely to involve co-offenders, who tended to be similar in age and sex to the Study males and lived close to their homes and to the locations of the offences. Violent offences were not particularly likely to involve co-offenders. The Study males were most likely to offend with brothers when they had brothers who were similar in age to them.

The major problem is whether young people are more likely to commit offences while they are in groups than while they are alone, or whether the high prevalence of co-offending merely reflects the fact that, whenever young people go out, they tend to go out in groups. Do peers tend to encourage and facilitate offending, or is it just that most kinds of activities out of the home (both delinquent and non-delinquent) tend to be performed in groups? Another possibility is that the commission of offences encourages association with other delinquents, perhaps because 'birds of a feather flock together' or because of the stigmatizing and isolating effects of court appearances and imprisonment. It is surprisingly difficult to decide among these various possibilities, although most researchers argue that peer influence is an important factor.

There is clearly a close relationship between the delinquent activities of a young person and those of his friends. Both in the United States and in England, it has been found that a boy's reports of his own offending are significantly correlated with his reports of his friends' delinquency. In the American National Youth Survey, having delinquent peers was the best independent predictor of self-reported offending in a multivariate analysis (Elliott *et al.* 1985). However, the major problem of interpretation is that, if delinquency is a group activity, delinquents will almost inevitably have delinquent friends, and this result does not necessarily show that delinquent friends cause offending.

Delinquent peers are likely to be most influential where they have high status within the peer group and are popular. However, studies both in the United States and in England show that delinquents are usually unpopular with their peers (Roff and Wirt, 1984). Indeed, aggressive children have been shown to be particularly likely to be rejected by their peers. It seems paradoxical for offending to be a group phenomenon facilitated by peer influence, and yet for offenders to be largely rejected by other adolescents. However, it may be that offenders are popular in antisocial groups and unpopular in prosocial groups.

School influences

It is clear that the prevalence of offending varies dramatically between different secondary schools (e.g. Power *et al.*, 1967). However, what is far less clear is how much of this variation should be attributed to differences in school climates and practices, and how much to differences in the composition of the student body.

In the Cambridge Study, the effects of secondary schools on offending was investigated by following boys from their primary schools to their secondary schools. The best primary-school predictor of convictions in this survey was the rating of troublesomeness at the age of 8–10 by peers and teachers. The secondary schools differed dramatically in their conviction rates, from one school with 20.9 court appearances per 100 boys per year to another where the corresponding figure was only 0.3. However, it was very noticeable that the most troublesome boys tended to go to the high-delinquency-rate schools, while the least troublesome boys tended to go to the low-delinquency-rate schools. Furthermore, it was clear that most of the variation between schools in their delinquency rates could be explained by differences in their intakes of troublesome boys. The secondary schools themselves had only a very small effect on the boys' offending.

The most famous study of school effects on offending was also carried out in Inner London by Rutter *et al.* (1979). Twelve comprehensive schools were studied, and big differences in official delinquency rates between them were found. High-delinquency-rate schools tended to have high truancy rates, low-ability pupils, and low-social-class parents. However, the differences between the schools in delinquency rates could not be entirely explained by differences in the social class and verbal reasoning scores of the pupils at intake (age 11). Therefore they must have been caused by some aspect of the schools themselves, or by other, unmeasured factors.

In trying to discover which aspects of schools might encourage or inhibit offending, a measure of 'school process' based on school structure, organization, and functioning was developed. This was related to school misbehaviour, academic achievement, and truancy. The main school factors that were related to offending were a high amount of punishment and a low amount of praise given by teachers in class. Unfortunately, it is difficult to know whether much punishment and little praise are causes or consequences of antisocial school behaviour, which in turn is probably linked to offending outside school.

Socio-economic deprivation

Most criminological theories assume that offenders disproportionally come from lower-class social backgrounds, and aim to explain why this is so. For example, it has been proposed by Cohen (1955) that lower-class boys find it hard to succeed according to the middle-class standards of the school, partly because lower-class parents tend not to teach their children to delay immediate gratification in favour of long-term goals. Consequently, lower-class boys join delinquent subcultures by whose standards they can succeed. It has been argued that lower-class children cannot achieve universal goals of status and material wealth by legitimate means, and consequently have to resort to offending.

Generally, the social class or socio-economic status of a family has been measured primarily according to rankings, by sociologists, of the occupational prestige of the family breadwinner. Persons with professional or managerial jobs are ranked in the highest class, while those with unskilled manual jobs are ranked in the lowest class. However, these occupational prestige scales may not correlate very highly with real differences between families in socio-economic circumstances. In general, the scales date from many years ago, when it was more common for the father to be the family breadwinner and for the mother to be a housewife. Because of this, it may be difficult to derive a realistic measure of socio-economic status for a family with a single parent or with two working parents.

Over the years, many other measures of social class have become popular, including family income, educational levels of parents, type of housing, overcrowding in the house, possessions, dependence on welfare benefits, and family size. These may all reflect more meaningful differences between families than occupational prestige. Family size is highly correlated with other indices of socio-economic deprivation, although its relationship with offending may reflect child-rearing factors (for instance less attention to each child) rather than socio-economic influences.

In the United States, it has been argued that low social class is related to arrests or convictions but not to self-reported offending, and hence that the official processing of offenders is biased against lower-class youth. However, English studies have reported more consistent links between low social class and offending. A national survey (Douglas *et al.*, 1966) has shown that the prevalence of juvenile convictions varies considerably according to the occupational prestige and educational background of the parents, from 3 per cent in the highest category to 19 per cent in the lowest. Also, it has been found that offending increases significantly with increasing family size. Similar results were reported in studies of Newcastle children from birth to the age of 33 (Kolvin *et al.*, 1988) and in Inner London (Ouston, 1984).

Numerous socio-economic indicators were measured in the Cambridge Study, both for the man's family of origin and for the man himself as an adult, including occupational prestige, family income, housing, employment instability, and family size. Most of the measures of occupational prestige (based on the Registrar General's scale) were not significantly related to offending. However, in a reversal of the American results, low social class of the family when the boy was aged 8–10 significantly predicted his later self-reported offending but not his convictions. More consistently, low family income, poor housing, and large family size predicted both convictions and self-reported offending. Low social class, low income, and large family size (but not poor housing) all predicted convictions for violence.

In research projects, socio-economic deprivation of parents is usually related to offending by sons. However, when the sons grow up, their own socio-economic deprivation can be related to their own offending. In the Cambridge Study, convicted and self-reported offenders tended to have unskilled manual jobs and an unstable job record at the age of 18. Also, between the ages of 15 and 18 the boys were convicted at a higher rate when they were unemployed than when they were employed, suggesting that unemployment in some way causes crime, and conversely that employment may lead to cessation of offending.

Community influences

Offending rates vary with area of residence. Studies in Chicago and other American cities (Shaw and McKay, 1969) showed that delinquency rates (based on where offenders lived) were highest in inner-city areas characterized by physical deterioration, neighbourhood disorganization, and high residential mobility. A large proportion of all offenders came from a small proportion of areas, which tended to be the most deprived. Furthermore, these relatively high delinquency rates persisted over time, despite the effect of successive waves of immigration and emigration in changing the population in different areas. Variations in offending rates reflected variations in the social values and norms to which children were exposed, which in turn reflected the degree of social disorganization of an area.

Later work has tended to cast doubt on the consistency of offending rates over time. More recent work in Chicago (Bursik and Webb, 1982) has shown that the distribution of offending was not stable after 1950, but reflected demographic changes. Variations in delinquency rates in different areas were significantly correlated with variations in the percentage of non-whites, the percentage of foreign-born whites, and the percentage of overcrowded households. The greatest increase in offending in an area occurred when blacks moved from the minority to the majority. These results suggested that Shaw and McKay's ideas, about community values which persisted despite successive waves of immigration and emigration, needed revising. It was necessary to take account both of the type of area and of the type of people living in the area.

Similar studies have been carried out in England. In London offending rates in one study (Wallis and Maliphant, 1967) correlated with rates of local-authority renting, the percentage of land used industrially or commercially, population density, overcrowded households, the proportion of non-white immigrants, and the proportion of the population aged under 21. A similar study was carried out in one working-class London borough by Power *et al.* (1972) and found that delinquency rates varied with rates of overcrowding and fertility and with the social class and type of housing in an area.

It is important to know why offending rates are higher in cities than in rural areas. One of the most important studies is a comparison of 10-year-old children in Inner London and the Isle of Wight (Rutter *et al.*, 1975*a*). A much higher incidence of conduct disorder was found in the Inner London sample. These results are relevant to delinquency, because of the link between conduct disorder in children and offending in juveniles and adults. Factors that might explain this area difference have been found to be family disorder, parental deviance, social disadvantages, and school characteristics. These were correlated with conduct disorder in each area, and it was concluded that the higher rates of disorder in Inner London were at least partly caused by the higher incidence of these four adverse factors.

A key question is why crime rates of communities change over time, and to what extent this is a function of changes in the communities or in the individuals living in them. Answering this question requires longitudinal research in which both communities and individuals are followed up. The best way of establishing the impact of the environment is to follow people who move from one area to another. In the Cambridge Study, it was found that moving out of London led to a significant decrease in convictions and self-reported offending, possibly because moving out led to a breaking up of offending groups. The differences between Inner London and the Isle of Wight held even when the analyses were restricted to children reared in the same area by parents reared in the same area. This suggests that the movement of problem families into problem areas cannot be the whole explanation of area differences in offending.

Clearly, there is an interaction between individuals and the communities in which they live. Some aspect of an inner city leads to a breakdown of community ties or neighbourhood patterns of mutual support; or perhaps the high population density produces tension, frustration, or anonymity. There may be interrelated factors. High-crime areas often have a high concentration of single-parent female-headed households with low incomes, living in low-cost, poor housing. The weakened parental control in these families – partly caused by the fact that the mother had to work and left her children unsupervised – meant that the children tended to congregate on the streets. In consequence, they were influenced by a peer subculture that often encourages offending.

Situational influences

While most criminological researchers have aimed to explain the development of offenders, some have tried to explain the occurrence of offending events. As has already been mentioned, offenders are predominantly versatile rather than specialized. Hence, in studying offenders, it seems unnecessary to develop a different theory for each different type of offender. In contrast, in trying to explain why offences occur, the situations are so diverse and specific to particular crimes that it probably is necessary to have different explanations for different types of offences.

The most popular theory of offending events suggests that they occur in response to specific opportunities, when their expected benefits (for example, stolen property, peer approval) outweigh their expected costs (for example legal punishment, parental disapproval). For example, a theory of residential burglary has been suggested (Clarke and Cornish, 1985) which included such influencing factors as whether a house was occupied, whether it looked affluent, whether there were bushes to hide behind, whether there were nosy neighbours, whether the house had a burglar alarm, and whether it contained a dog. It has been proposed that offending involves a rational decision in which expected benefits are weighed against expected costs.

In the Cambridge Study, the most common reasons given for offending were rational ones, suggesting that most property crimes were committed because the offenders wanted to steal the items. Also, a number of surveys have shown that low estimates of the risk of being caught are correlated with high rates of self-reported offending. Unfortunately, the direction of causal influence is not clear in these studies, since committing offences may lead to lower estimates of the probability of detection as well as the reverse. However, it is plausible to suggest that opportunities for offending, the immediate costs and benefits of offending, and the probabilities of these outcomes, all influence whether people offend in any situation.

Explaining crime

One of the greatest problems in interpreting results is that causal factors tend to be related to each other. People living in high-crime areas tend to be socio-economically deprived, tend to use erratic methods of child-rearing and to have poor supervision, tend to have children who are impulsive and who have low school attainment, and so on. The explanation, prevention, and treatment of offending requires some disentangling of the mass of interrelations; but this is very difficult to achieve convincingly.

A first step is to establish which factors predict offending independently of other factors. In the Cambridge Study, it was generally true that each group of influences (for example family influence or school problems) predicted offending independently of every other. The independent predictors of convictions between the ages of 10 and 20 included troublesomeness, convicted parents, high daring, low school attainment, poor housing, and poor parental child-rearing. Hence it might be concluded that antisocial influences, impulsivity, school problems, socio-economic deprivation, and family factors, despite their interplay, all contribute independently to the development of offending.

David Farrington's theory proposes that the major factors fostering antisocial tendencies are impulsivity, a poor ability to manipulate abstract concepts, low empathy, a weak conscience, internalized norms and attitudes favouring offending, and long-term motivating influences such as the desire for material goods or status with peers. The major factors that influence whether antisocial tendencies are translated into crimes are short-term situational factors such as boredom, frustration, alcohol consumption, opportunities to offend, and the perceived costs and benefits of offending.

PREVENTION AND TREATMENT

Methods of preventing or treating offending should be based on causes. Implications about prevention and treatment from some of the likely causes of offending listed above will now be drawn. The methods reviewed here are those for which there is some scientific justification.

Skills training

Attempts have been made to change impulsivity and other personality characteristics of offenders using the set of techniques variously termed 'cognitive – behavioural interpersonal social skills training' or some subset of those labels. For example, some methods of treating juvenile delinquents are solidly based on some of the known individual characteristics of offenders: their impulsivity, poor abstract reasoning, egocentricity, and poor interpersonal problem-solving skills.

It has been argued that delinquents can be taught the cognitive skills in which they are deficient, and that this can lead to a decrease in their offending. Reviews of delinquency-rehabilitation programmes show that those which have been successful in reducing crime have generally tried to change the offender's thinking. A 'Reasoning and Rehabilitation' programme has been carried out in Canada, and led to a significant decrease in reoffending. Training was carried out by probation officers, although it was of a kind that might also have been administered by parents and teachers (Ross *et al.*, 1988).

This programme aimed to teach delinquents to stop and think before acting, to consider the consequences of their behaviour, to conceptualize alternative ways of solving interpersonal problems, and to consider the impact of their behaviour on other people, especially their victims. It included social skills training, lateral thinking (to teach creative problem-solving), critical thinking (to teach logical reasoning), value education (to teach values and concern for others), assertiveness training (to teach non-aggressive, socially appropriate ways to obtain desired outcomes), negotiation-skills training, interpersonal cognitive problem-solving (to teach thinking skills for solving interpersonal problems), social perspective training (to teach how to recognize and understand other people's feelings), and role-playing and modelling (demonstration and practice of effective and acceptable interpersonal behaviour).

Parent-training

If poor parental supervision and erratic child-rearing behaviour are causes of offending, it seems likely that parent training might succeed in reducing offending. Behavioural parent training is one of the most hopeful approaches (Patterson, 1982). Careful observations of parent-child interaction have shown that parents of antisocial children are deficient in their methods of child-rearing. These parents fail to tell their children how they are expected to behave, fail to monitor the behaviour to ensure that it is desirable, and fail to enforce rules promptly and unambiguously with appropriate rewards and penalties. The parents of antisocial children use more punishment (such as scolding, shouting, or threatening), but fail to make it contingent on the child's behaviour.

Attempts have been made to train these parents in effective child-rearing methods, namely noticing what a child is doing, monitoring behaviour over long periods, clearly stating house rules, making rewards and punishments contingent on behaviour, and negotiating disagreements so that conflicts and crises do not escalate. This treatment has been shown to be effective in reducing child stealing. Parent training is often effective in reducing childhood aggression and conduct disorder, but is most successful with two harmonious parents (Kazdin, 1985).

Peer and school programmes

Several studies show that school children can be taught to resist peer influences encouraging smoking, drinking, and marijuana use. For example, older high-school students have been employed to teach younger ones to develop counter-arguing skills to resist peer pressure to smoke. This approach was successful in decreasing smoking by the younger students (Telch *et al.*, 1982). Same-aged peer leaders (children with high prestige) have been used to teach students how to resist peer pressures to begin smoking, again with successful results. These techniques, designed to counter antisocial peer pressures, could be used to decrease offending.

If low intelligence and school problems are causes of offending, then any programme that leads to an increase in school success should lead to a decrease in offending. One of the most successful delinquency-prevention programmes was the Perry pre-school project carried out in Michigan. This was targeted on disadvantaged black children, who were allocated (approximately at random) to experimental and control groups. The experimental children attended a daily pre-school programme, backed up by weekly home visits, usually lasting two years (covering ages 3–4). The aim of the programme was to provide intellectual stimulation, to increase cognitive abilities, and to increase later school achievement.

More than 120 children were followed up to the age of 15, using teacher ratings, parent and youth interviews, and school records. As has been demonstrated in several other similar projects, the experimental group showed gains in intelligence that were rather short-lived. However, they were significantly better in elementary school motivation, school achievement at the age of 14, teacher ratings of classroom behaviour at 6 to 9, self-reports of classroom behaviour at 15, and self-reports of offending at 15. Furthermore, a later follow-up showed that, at the age of 19, the experimental group was more likely to be employed, more likely to have graduated from high school, more likely to have received college or vocational training, and less likely to have been arrested (Berrueta-Clement *et al.*, 1984). Hence, this pre-school intellectual enrichment programme led to decreases in school failure and to decreases in offending.

A programme intended to decrease aggressive behaviour, delinquency, and drug-abuse, and to increase socially acceptable behaviour, by promoting social bonding has been carried out by Hawkins *et al.* (1991). About 500 first-grade children (aged 6) in eight Seattle schools were randomly assigned to be in experimental or control classes. The children in the experimental classes received special treatment at home and school which was designed to increased their attachment to their parents and their bonding to the school. Their parents were trained to notice and reinforce socially desirable behaviour in a programme called 'Catch 'em being good'. Their teachers were trained in classroom-management, for example to provide clear instructions and expectations to children, to reward children for participation in desired behaviour, and to teach children socially acceptable methods of solving problems.

In an evaluation of this programme 18 months later, when the children were in different classes, boys who received the experimental programme were significantly less aggressive than the control boys, according to teacher ratings. This difference was particularly marked for white boys rather than black boys. Girls were not significantly less aggressive, but they were less self-destructive, anxious, and depressed.

A large-scale programme designed to reduce bullying in Norwegian schools has been carried out by Olweus (1991). The programme was targeted on teachers, parents, and children in schools containing children aged 8–16. A booklet was distributed to all schools describing what was known about bullying and what steps schools and teachers could take to reduce it. Simultaneously, the schools distributed to all parents a folder containing information and advice about bullying. The main aims of the programme were to increase awareness and knowledge of bullying, to increase active involvement by teachers, parents, and children in preventing bullying, and to increase support for victims of bullying by other children. In addition, teachers developed clear rules against bullying and applied consistent sanctions against bullies, and the monitoring and supervision of children by adults (especially in the playground) was improved.

The success of the programme in 42 schools in Bergen has been evaluated using before and after measures (self-reports of bullying and being bullied). The programme was successful in reducing the incidence of bullying by half. A similar programme is currently being implemented in Sheffield.

Situational crime prevention

A number of crime-prevention methods have been based on situational influences on crime and have been shown to be effective. These methods are typically aimed at specific types of offences, and are designed to change the environment to decrease criminal opportunities. They include increasing surveillance (for example, by installing closed-circuit television cameras in underground stations), hardening targets (for example, by replacing aluminium coin boxes by steel ones in public telephone kiosks), and managing the environment (for example, by paying wages by cheque rather than by cash).

The major difficulty with this approach is that if some people have criminal propensities, and one outlet for these is blocked, they will seek other outlets: other types of crimes, other methods of committing crimes, other targets, and so on. Also, situational approaches provoke fears of 'big brother' forms of state control and of a 'fortress society' in which frightened citizens scuttle from their fortified house, in their fortified car, to their fortified workplace, avoiding contact with other citizens. This kind of approach is obviously counterproductive in the management of patients; and it is unfortunate that some casualty departments resemble Fort Knox. Nevertheless, situational crime prevention is clearly an important approach which holds out the promise of decreasing offending.

If offending involves a rational decision in which the costs are weighed against the benefits, it might be deterred by increasing the costs of offending or by increasing their probability. Indeed, research on the effect of the breathalyser on drunken driving and on the effect of arresting men for domestic violence suggests that adults can be deterred (Ross *et al.*, 1970; Sherman and Berk, 1984). However, the attempt to deter juveniles in the 'Scared Straight' programme, by having adult prisoners tell then about the horrors of imprisonment, was not successful (Finckenauer, 1982). Given the 'macho' orientation of many young offenders, it may be that these warnings made offending seem more risky and hence more attractive.

SUMMARY

Generally, offending is versatile, since people who commit one type of crime tend also to commit other types. Violent offenders tend to be frequent and persistent offenders. Hence, the causes of violence are essentially the same as the causes of frequent and persistent antisocial and criminal behaviour. Offending is only one element of a larger syndrome of antisocial behaviour which arises in childhood and usually persists into adulthood. Research is needed on how to protect children from criminogenic backgrounds from developing this syndrome.

Offending peaks in the teenage years, although violent offending tends to peak a little later. Generally, males offend more than females, and blacks offend more than whites, who in turn offend more than Asians (at least in England). There may be some genetic influences on crime. Offenders tend to have a fearless and uninhibited childhood temperament, have low arousal, and are impulsive. They also tend to have low intelligence and low achievement at school. Their parents tend to be antisocial and criminal, and to use physical abuse, harsh and erratic discipline, and poor supervision. Offenders tend to be separated from their natural parents for reasons other than death or hospitalization. They tend to come from economically deprived families, to have delinquent friends, to attend delinquent schools, and to live in deprived areas. Offending seems to involve a cost – benefit decision.

Possible methods of preventing offending include social skills training, parent training, using prosocial peer influences, pre-school intellectual enrichment programmes, and situational crime prevention. It is clear that any measure that succeeds in reducing offending will have wide-ranging benefits. Any measure that reduces offending will probably also reduce alcohol-abuse, drunk driving, drug-abuse, sexual promiscuity, family violence, truancy, school failure, unemployment, marital disharmony, and divorce. It is clear that antisocial children tend to grow up into antisocial adults, and that antisocial adults tend to produce more antisocial children. Major efforts to tackle the problems of antisocial personality, offending, and violence, which pose major threats to public health, are urgently needed.

FURTHER READING

Eysenck, H.J. and Gudjonsson, G.H. (1989). *The causes and cures of criminality. Plenum, New York.*

Farrington, D. P., Berkowitz, L., and West, D. J. (1982). Differences between individual and group fights. *British Journal of Social Psychology*, **21**, 323–33.

Farrington, D.P., Ohlin, L.E., and Wilson, J.Q. (1986). *Understanding and controlling crime.* Springer-Verlag, New York.

Farrington, D.P. and West, D.J. (1990). The Cambridge Study in delinquent development: a long-term follow-up of 411 London males. In *Criminality: personality, behaviour, and life history*, H.J. Kerner and G. Kaiser, (eds) pp. 115–38. Springer-Verlag, Berlin.

Kazdin, A.E. (1985). *Treatment of antisocial behaviour in children and adolescents.* Dorsey, Homewood, Illinois.

Pepler, D.J. and Rubin, K.H. (eds) (1991). *The development and treatment of childhood aggression.* Erlbaum, Hillsdale, New Jersey.

Rutter, M. and Giller, H. (1983). *Juvenile delinquency.* Penguin, Harmondsworth.

West, D.J. (1969). *Present conduct and future delinquency.* Heinemann, London.

West, D.J. (1982). *Delinquency: its roots, careers and prospects.* Heinemann, London.

Wilson, J.Q. and Herrnstein, R.J. (1985). *Crime and human nature.* Simon and Schuster, New York.

REFERENCES

Berrueta-Clement, J.R., Schweinhart, L.J., Barnett, W.S., Epstein, A.S., and Weikart, D.P. (1984). *Changed lives.* Ypsilanti, Michigan: High/Scope.

Bouchard, T.J., Lykken, D.T., McGue, M., Segal, N.L., and Tellegen, A. (1990). Sources of human psychological differences: The Minnesota study of twins reared apart. *Science*, **250**, 223–8.

Bursik, R.J. and Webb, J. (1982). Community change and patterns of delinquency. *American Journal of Sociology*, **88**, 24–42.

Campbell, A. (1981). *Girl delinquents.* Blackwell, Oxford.

Clarke, R.V. and Cornish, D.B. (1985). Modelling offenders' decisions: A framework for research and policy. *In* M. Tonry and N. Morris (ed.) *Crime and Justice*, vol. 6, pp. 147–85. University of Chicago Press, Chicago.

Cohen, A.K. (1955). *Delinquent boys.* Free Press, Glencoe, Illinois.

Douglas, J.W.B., Ross, J.M., Hammond, W.A., and Mulligan, D.G. (1966). Delinquency and social class. *British Journal of Criminology*, **6**, 294–302.

Elliott, D.S., Huizinga, D., and Ageton, S.S. (1985). *Explaining delinquency and drug use.* Sage, Beverly Hills, California.

Eysenck, H.J. (1977). *Crime and personality* (3rd edn.). Routledge and Kegan Paul, London.

Eysenck, H.J. and Gudjonsson, G.H. (1989). *The causes and cures of criminality.* Plenum, New York.

Farrington, D.P. (1986). Age and crime. *In* M. Tonry and N. Morris (ed.) *Crime and justice*, vol. 7 pp. 189–250. University of Chicago Press, Chicago.

Farrington, D.P. (1992). Juvenile delinquency. *In* J.C. Coleman (ed.) *The school years* (2nd edn), (pp. 123–63). Routledge, London.

Farrington, D.P., Berkowitz, L., and West, D.J. (1982*a*). Differences between individual and group fights. *British Journal of Social Psychology*, **21**, 323–33.

Farrington, D.P., Biron, L., and LeBlanc, M. (1982*b*). Personality and delinquency in London and Montreal. *In* J. Gunn and D.P. Farrington (ed.). *Abnormal offenders, delinquency, and the criminal justice system*, pp. 153–201. Wiley, Chichester.

Farrington, D.P., Loeber, R., and Van Kammen, W.B. (1990). Long-term criminal outcomes of hyperactivity-impulsivity – attention deficit and conduct problems in childhood. *In* L.N. Robins and M. Rutter (eds). *Straight and devious pathways from childhood to adulthood* (pp. 62–81). Cambridge University Press.

Farrington, D.P. and West, D.J. (1990). The Cambridge study in delinquent development: A long-term follow-up of 411 London males. *In* H.J. Kerner and G. Kaiser (ed.) *Criminality: personality, behaviour, life history* (pp. 115–38). Springer-Verlag, Berlin.

Finckenauer, J.O. (1982). *Scared straight.* Prentice-Hall, Englewood Cliffs, N.J.

Gordon, R.A. (1987). SES versus IQ in the race-IQ-delinquency model. *International Journal of Sociology and Social Policy*, 7, 30–96.

Gottfredson, M. and Hirschi, T. (1990). *A general theory of crime.* Stanford University Press, California.

Gove, W.R. (1985). The effect of age and gender on deviant behaviour: A biopsychosocial perspective. *In* A.S. Rossi (ed.) *Gender and the life course* (pp. 115–44). Aldine, Hawthorne, N.Y.

Hawkins, J.D., Von Cleve, E., and Catalano, R.F. (1991). Reducing early childhood aggression: results of a primary prevention programme. *Journal of the American Academy of Child and Adolescent Psychiatry*, 30, 208–17.

Home Office (1993). *Criminal statistics, England and Wales, 1991.* Her Majesty's Stationery Office, London.

Home Office Statistical Bulletin (1989a). *Crime statistics for the Metropolitan Police District by ethnic group, 1987: victims, suspects and those arrested.* Home Office, London.

Home Office Statistical Bulletin (1989b). *Criminal and custodial careers of those born in 1953, 1958, and 1963.* Home Office, London.

Kagan, J., Reznick, J.S., and Snidman, N. (1988). Biological bases of childhood shyness. *Science*, 240, 167–71.

Kandel, E. and Mednick, S.A. (1991). Perinatal complications predict violent offending. *Criminology*, 29, 519–29.

Kazdin, A.E. (1985). *Treatment of antisocial behaviour in children and adolescents.* Dorsey Press, Homewood, Illinois.

Kolvin, I., Miller, F.J.W., Fleeting, M., and Kolvin, P.A. (1988). Social and parenting factors affecting criminal-offence rates: findings from the Newcastle Thousand Family Study (1947–1980). *British Journal of Psychiatry*, 152, 80–90.

Loeber, R. and Dishion, T. (1983). Early predictors of male delinquency: a review. *Psychological Bulletin*, 94, 68–99.

Loeber, R. and Stouthamer-Loeber, M. (1983). Family factors as correlates and predictors of juvenile conduct problems and delinquency. *In* M. Tonry and N. Morris (ed.) *Crime and justice*, vol. 7 (pp. 29–149). University of Chicago Press, Chicago.

Maccoby, E.E. and Jacklin, C.N. (1974). *The psychology of sex differences.* Stanford University Press, California.

Magnusson, D. (1988). *Individual development from an interactional perspective.* Erlbaum, Hillsdale, N.J.

Mawby, R.I., McCulloch, J.W. and Batta, I.D. (1979). Crime amongst Asian juveniles in Bradford. *International Journal of the sociology of Law*, 7, 297–306.

Mawson, A.R. (1987). *Transient criminality.* Praeger, New York.

Mayhew, P., Elliott, D., and Dowds, L. (1989). *The 1988 British crime survey.* H.M.S.O., London.

Mednick, S.A., Gabrielli, W.F., and Hutchings, B. (1983). Genetic influences on criminal behaviour: evidence from an adoption cohort. *In* K.T. Van Dusen and S.A. Mednick (ed.) *Prospective studies of crime and delinquency* (pp. 39–56). Kluwer-Nijhoff, Boston.

Moffitt, T.E. and Silva, P.A. (1988). Neuropsychological deficit and self-reported delinquency in an unselected birth cohort. *Journal of the American Academy of Child and Adolescent Psychiatry*, **27**, 233–40.

Olweus, D. (1987). Testosterone and adrenaline: aggressive antisocial behaviour in normal adolescent males. *In* S.A. Mednick, T.E. Moffitt, and S.A. Stack (ed.) *The causes of crime: new biological approaches* (pp. 263–82). Cambridge University Press.

Olweus, D. (1991). Bully/victim problems among schoolchildren. *In* Pepler, D.J. and Rubin, K.H. (ed.) *The development and treatment of childhood aggression* (pp. 411–48). Erlbaum, Hillsdale, N.J.

Ouston, J. (1984). Delinquency, family background, and educational attainment. *British Journal of Criminology*, **24**, 2–26.

Patterson, G.R. (1982). *Coercive family process*. Castalia, Eugene, Oregon.

Pepler, D.J. and Rubin, K.H. (1991). (ed.). *The development and treatment of childhood aggression*. Erlbaum. Hillsdale, N.J.

Power, M.J., Alderson, M.R., Phillipson, C.M., Shoenberg, E., and Morris, J.N. (1967). Delinquent schools? *New Society*, **10**, 542–3.

Power, M.J., Benn, R.T., and Morris, J.N. (1972). Neighbourhood, schools, and juveniles before the courts. *British Journal of Criminology*, **12**, 111–32.

Reiss, A.J. and Farrington, D.P. (1991). Advancing knowledge about co-offending: results from a prospective longitudinal survey of London males. *Journal of Criminal Law and Criminology*, **82**, 360–95.

Riley, D. and Shaw, M. (1985). *Parental supervision and juvenile delinquency*. HMSO, London.

Roff, J.D. and Wirt, R.D. (1984). Childhood aggression and social adjustment as antecedents of delinquency. *Journal of Abnormal Child Psychology*, **12**, 111–26.

Ross, H.L., Campbell, D.T., and Glass, G.V. (1970). Determining the social effects of a legal reform: the British breathalyzer crackdown of 1967. *American Behavioural Scientist*, **13**, 493–509.

Ross, R.R., Fabiano, E.A., and Ewles, C.D. (1988). Reasoning and rehabilitation. *International Journal of Offender Therapy and Comparative Criminology*, **32**, 29–35.

Rutter, M., Cox, A., Tupling, C., Berger, M., and Yule, W. (1975a). Attainment and adjustment in two geographical areas: I. The prevalence of psychiatric disorder. *British Journal of Psychiatry*, **126**, 493–509.

Rutter, M. and Giller, H. (1983). *Juvenile delinquency.*, Penguin, Harmondsworth.

Rutter, M., Maughan, B., Mortimore, P., and Ouston, J. (1979). *Fifteen thousand hours*. Open Books, London.

Rutter, M., Yule, B., Quinton, D., Rowlands, O., Yule, W., and Berger, M. (1975b) Attainment and adjustment in two geographical areas: III. Some factors accounting for area differences. *British Journal of Psychiatry*, **126**, 520–33.

Shaw, C.R. and McKay, H.D. (1969). Juvenile delinquency and urban areas (revised ed.). University of Chicago Press, Chicago.

Sherman, L.W. and Berk, R.A. (1984). The specific deterrent effects of arrest for domestic assault. *American Sociological Review*, **49**, 261–72.

Telch, M.J., Killen, J.D., McAlister, A.L., Perry, C.L. and Maccoby, N. (1982). Long-term follow-up of a pilot project on smoking prevention with adolescents. *Journal of Behavioural Medicine*, **5**, 1–8.

Tonry, M., Ohlin, L.E., and Farrington, D.P. (1991). *Human development and criminal behaviour*. Springer-Verlag, New York.

Tracy, P.E., Wolfgang, M.E., and Figlio, R.M. (1985). *Delinquency in two birth cohorts*. National Institute of Juvenile Justice and Delinquency Prevention, Washington, DC.

Venables, P.H., and Raine, A. (1987). Biological theory. *In* B.J. McGurk, D.M. Thornton, and M. Williams (ed.). *Applying psychology to imprisonment* (pp. 3–27). HMSO, London.

Visher, C.A. and Roth, J.A. (1986). Participation in criminal careers. In A. Blumstein, J. Cohen, J.A. Roth, and C.A. Visher (ed.). *Criminal careers and 'career criminals'*, vol. 1 (pp. 211–91). National Academy Press, Washington, DC.

Wadsworth, M. (1979). *Roots of delinquency*. Martin Robertson, London.

Wallis, C.P. and Maliphant, R. (1967). Delinquent areas in the county of London: ecological factors. *British Journal of Criminology*, **7**, 250–84.

Widom, C.S. (1989). The cycle of violence. *Science*, **244**, 160–6.

Wilson, H. (1980). Parental supervision: a neglected aspect of delinquency. *British Journal of Criminology*, **20**, 203–35.

Wilson, J.Q. and Herrnstein, R.J. (1985). *Crime and human nature*. Simon and Schuster, New York.

Wolfgang, M.E., Thornberry, T.P., and Figlio, R.M. (1987). *From boy to man, from delinquency to crime*. University of Chicago Press, Chicago.

Association of University Teachers
(AUT)
9 Pembridge Road
LONDON
W11 3JY
TEL: 071 221 4370

Provides legal and
contractual advice.

Association of British Dental Surgery
Assistants (ABDSA)
DSA House
29 London Street
FLEETWOOD
Lancashire
SY7 6JY
TEL: 0253 778631

Provides emotional support
through local co-ordinators.
Advises on sources of legal
aid (for example, Citizens' Advice
Bureau).

British Association of Applied
Chiropractic (BAAC)
The Old Post Office
Stratton Audley
BICESTER
OX6 9BA
TEL: 0869 277111

Membership benefits,
including legal advice.

British Association of Occupational
Therapists (BAOT)
6/8 Marshalsea Road
LONDON
SE1 1HL
TEL: 071 357 6480

Publishes guidelines on
dealing with violent
behaviour. Membership
benefits include personal
injury insurance. Advises on
contractual and legal
problems.

British Association of Social Workers
(BASW)
16 Kent Street
BIRMINGHAM
B5 6RD
TEL: 021 622 3911

Membership benefits
include personal injury and
clothing insurance.
Encourages staff care and
'buddy' support services.
Provides representation of
members in discussions and
negotiations with
employers. Publishes book
Social workers at risk.

British Dental Association (BDA)
64 Wimpole Street
LONDON
W1M 8AL
TEL: 071 935 0875

Advises on loss of earnings and contractual and legal problems. Advises on security. Refers members to Medical Defence organizations.

British Dental Hygienists Association (BDHA)
64 Wimpole Street
LONDON
W1M 8AL
TEL: 0934 833932

Advises on sources of legal assistance.

British Dietetic Association (BDA)
7th Floor, Elizabeth House
22 Suffolk Street Queensway
BIRMINGHAM
B1 1LS
TEL: 021 643 5483

Provides counselling from Industrial Liaison Officers. Gives legal advice from BDA solicitors.

British Medical Association (BMA)
British Medical Association House
Tavistock Square
LONDON
WC1H 9JP
TEL: 071 387 4499

Refers members to Regional Industrial Liaison Officers. Gives assistance with contractual and legal problems. Refers enquirers to Medical Defence organizations.

British Orthoptic Society (BOS)
Tavistock House North
Tavistock Square
LONDON
WC1H 9HX
TEL: 071 387 7992

Provides representation in discussions/disputes with employers.

British Psychological Society (BPS)
St Andrews House
48 Princess Road East
LEICESTER
LE1 7DR
TEL: 0533 549568

Makes grants from welfare fund in some cases. Advises on sources of legal help. See also under MSF. Refers psychologists with a role in education to either the National Union of Teachers or the Association of Educational Psychologists.

British Union of Social Work Employees (BUSWE)
BUSWE House
208 Middleton Road
Crumpsall
MANCHESTER
M8 4NA
TEL: 061 720 7727

Provides legal advice and representation in discussions with employers. Commnicates with police on behalf of members.

Chartered Society of Physiotherapy (CSP)
14 Bedford Row
LONDON
WC1R 4ED
TEL: 071 242 1941

Gives free legal advice from CSP Solicitors. Refers members to Medical Defence organizations. Provides guidance packs on safety to Community Physiotherapists.

College of Speech and Language Therapists (CSLT)
7 Bath Place
Rivington Street
LONDON
EC2A 3DR
TEL: 071 613 3855

Refers enquirers to appropriate Trade Union. For support services for Speech and Language Therapists see under MSF.

Confederation of Health Service Employees (COHSE)
Glen House
High Street
Banstead
Surrey
SM7 2LH
TEL: 0737 353322

Refers members to Regional Offices. Gives legal advice. Publishes comprehensive information packs 'Violence to staff in the Health Services' and 'Preventing violence to staff.' Provides representation in legal/ contractual negotiations. Ensures employers meet obligations in relation to prevention and recording of incidents.

NB: Merged with NUPE and NALGO to form 'UNISON' in 1993.

Employing Authorities (Self-Governing Trusts and Health Authorities)

Hospital Services

Provide Nursing/Junior Medical Staff Counsellors and Occupational Health/Personnel/Legal Departments. Advise on criminal/police procedures. Formal guidelines on safety/management of aggressive patients available in some Trusts/ Health Authorities.

Community Services	As for hospital services, but free personal alarms are provided for all staff in some Trusts. Portable telephones provided for staff in high-risk areas. Advice available from Security Officers. Training courses on handling aggression and self-defence and staff counsellors are provided by some authorities.
Guild of Hospital Pharmacists (GHP)	See under MSF.
Health and Safety Commission (HSC) (Health Services Advisory Committee) Baynards House 1 Chepstow Place LONDON W2 4TF TEL: 071 243 6630	Produces annual statistics on *Accident, injury, and ill-health.* Employers are required under 'Reporting, of Injuries, Diseases and Dangerous Occurrences' (RIDDOR) regulations to report incidents resulting in more than 3 days' incapacity. HSC or District Councils advise employers on injury prevention through area offices. Publishes *Preventing Violence to staff.* Area officers approach employers to ensure that appropriate staff training in prevention is being given and also that services for victims (for example, counselling services) are available.
Health Visitors Association (HVA) 50 Southwark Street LONDON SE1 1UN TEL: 071 378 7255	Ensures that incidents are recorded by employers and/or at premises where assaults took place. Arranges contact with local HVA representatives. Publishes guidelines on *Violence at work* and *Working alone.* Membership benefits include personal injury insurance. Gives legal/ contractual advice. Local representatives advise employers.
Institute of Medical Laboratory Sciences (IMLS) 12 Queen Anne Street LONDON W1M 0AU TEL: 071 636 8192	Refers enquirers to employing authorities. Runs 'legal helpline'.

Institute of Pure Chiropractic (IPC)
14 Park End Street
OXFORD
OX1 1HH
TEL: 0865 246687

Membership benefits include legal advice.

Manufacturing, Science and Finance (MSF) (formerly Association of Scientific, Technical and Managerial Staff (ASTMS) and Technical and Supervisory Staff (TASS)
Park House
64–6 Wandsworth Common
North Side
LONDON
SW18 2SH
TEL: 081 871 2100

Publishes booklet *Working Alone* for Community staff. Produces model agreement for measures to promote safety at work. Provides legal advice and representation in discussions with employing authorities and in the courts.

Medical Defence Union (MDU)
3 Devonshire Place
LONDON
W1N 2EA
TEL: 071 486 6181

Membership open to broad spectrum of health-care workers. Membership benefits include personal injury insurance. Advises on CICB claims, civil claims, criminal procedures.

Medical Protection Society (MPS)
50 Hallam Street
LONDON
W1N 6DE
TEL: 071 637 0541

Membership open to broad spectrum of health-care workers. Membership benefits include injury insurance. Advises on CICB claims, civil claims, criminal procedures.

National Association of Local Government Officials (NALGO)
1 Mabledon Place
LONDON
WC1H 9AJ
TEL: 071 388 2366

Publishes booklets on violence prevention. Refers victims to local branch secretary. Liaises with employers concerning recording and prevention of injury. Ensures that employers provide adequate counselling services, including those for relatives of deceased members (consistent with the recommendations of the 'Skelmersdale' DHSS Committee *Violence to staff* report, 1988). Ensures that employers investigate incidents so that prevention measures can be instituted. Helps with legal advice and compensation claims.

NB: Merged with COHSE and NUPE to form 'UNISON' in 1993.

National Union of Public Employees (NUPE)
Civic House
20 Grand Depot Road
Woolwich
LONDON
SE18 6SF
TEL: 081 854 2244

Publishes booklet *Violence in the NHS*. Gives legal advice. Health and and Safety Officers give advice. Provides representation in legal/contractual negotiations. Ensures employers meet obligations in relation to prevention of violence and recording of incidents.

NB: Merged with COHSE and NALGO to form 'UNISON' in 1993.

National Union of Students (NUS)
461 Holloway Road
LONDON
N7 6LJ
TEL: 071 272 8900

Refers victims to Welfare Officers. Women's Officers at particular schools, colleges, and universities. Welfare officers refer victims to counsellors (salaried posts: most are psychologists). Liaises with college authorities, such as Deans. Arranges legal aid certificates and liaises with solicitors regarding civil/criminal proceedings.

National Pharmaceutical Association (NPA)
38–42 St Peters Street
ST ALBANS
AL1 3NP
TEL: 0727 832161

Provides legal advice. Monthly supplement circulated to all members which includes features on violence and threatened violence. Advises on CICB claims. Dedicated insurance arrangements for Pharmacists in respect of premises, contents, and hold-ups.

Osteopathic Association of Great Britain (OAGB)
206 Chesterton Road
CAMBRIDGE
CB4 1NE
TEL: 0223 359236

Provides legal advice. Legal 'helpline' services purchased by OAGB. Arranges informal support for colleagues.

Royal College of Midwives (RCM)
15 Mansfield Street
LONDON
W1M OBE
TEL: 071 637 8823

Liaises with employing authorities about escorts and drivers for Community Midwives and about other safety aspects. Membership benefits include personal injury insurance.

Royal College of Nursing (RCN) 20 Cavendish Square LONDON W1M OAB TEL: 071 409 3333	Refers enquirers to regional offices. Helps with CICB applications and police investigations. Individual counselling by RCN stewards (personal support). Publishes leaflets on the management of aggression.
Royal Pharmaceutical Society of Great Britain (RPSGB) 1 Lambeth High Street LONDON SE1 7JN TEL: 071 735 9141	Makes grants from benevolent fund in some cases. Runs 'Birdsgrove House' (Convalescent Home). RPSGB Regional Inspectors advise on security issues. 'Sick Pharmacists Scheme' in development. Emotional support available from benevolent fund staff.
Society of Chiropodists and Podiatrists (SCP) 53 Welbeck Street LONDON W1M 7HE TEL: 071 486 3381	Negotiates enhanced salary levels for staff working in high-risk areas (for example in Psychiatric Units). Gives legal advice. Publishes *Minimum conditions of service*. Refers enquirers to the Department of Health Publication: *Violence to staff*.
Society of Radiographers 14 Upper Wimpole Street LONDON W1M 8BN TEL: 071 935 5726	Provides legal advice.
Social Care Association (SCA) 23a Victoria Road SURBITON Surrey KT6 4JZ TEL: 081 390 6831	Carries out continuous negotiations with local authorities, charities, and private residential homes and schools, particularly in relation to staffing levels. Membership benefits include personal injury cover. Advises and represents members (mostly care staff in residential homes) concerning 'good practice', which includes dealing with violent/aggressive behaviour. Provides 'legal helpline' and emotional support from local officers.

Transport and General Workers Union (TGWU)
Transport House
Smith Square
LONDON
SW1P 3JB
TEL: 071 828 7788

Provides legal support and representation. Negotiates with employers at national and local level. Helps with compensation claims.

Trades Union Congress (TUC)
Congress House
23–8 Great Russell Street
LONDON
WC1B 3LS
TEL: 071 636 4030

Publishes booklet *Violence to staff*. Publishes book *Hazards at work*. Co-ordinates and initiates Trade Union policy on safety. Provides training for Safety Representatives of Trade Unions.

UNISON
Unison Centre
Holborn Tower,
137–44 High Holborn,
LONDON
WC1V 6PL
TEL: 071 404 1884

See under COHSE, NUPE and NALGO

APPENDIX II: Other useful addresses and telephone numbers

Criminal Injuries Compensation Authority (CICA)
Tay House
300 Bath Street
GLASGOW
G2 4JR
TEL: 041 331 2726

National Counselling Service for Sick Doctors
1 Park Square West
LONDON
NW1 4LJ
TEL: 071 935 5982

Victim Support
Cranmer House
39 Brixton Road
LONDON SW9 62Z
TEL: 071 735 9166

Women's Aid National Helpline
PO BOX 391
BRISTOL
BS99 7WS
TEL: 0272 633542

INDEX